PLAY HELPS

22.99 Learning Centre

Coldharbour Lane, Hayes, Middlesex UB3 3BB
01895 853740 (Voice) / 01895 853661 (Minicom)

UXBRIDGE
COLLEGE

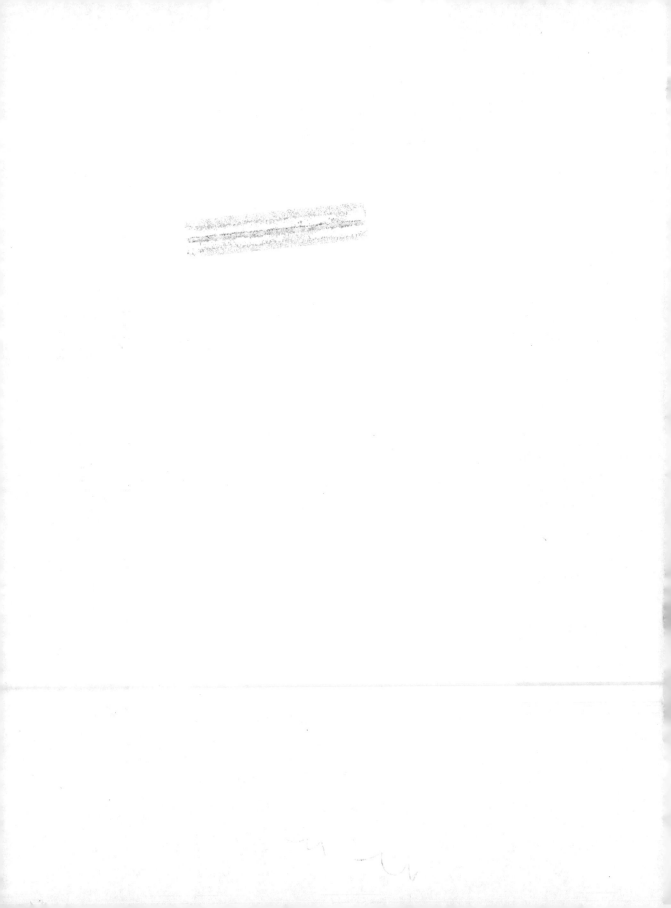

PLAY HELPS

Toys and Activities for Children with Special Needs

Fourth Edition

Roma Lear

Illustrated by Jill Hunter

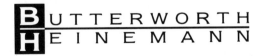

BUTTERWORTH
HEINEMANN

Butterworth-Heinemann
An imprint of Elsevier Limited

First published 1977
Second edition 1986
Third edition 1993
Fourth edition 1996
      Reprinted 1997, 1998, 2000, 2003, 2005

ISBN 0 7506 2522 8

British Library Cataloguing in Publication Data
Lear, Roma
    Play helps: toys and activities for children with special needs – 4th ed.
    1. Play therapy   2. Sick children – Recreation   3. Handicapped
    children – Recreation   4. Amusements
    I. Title   II. Hunter, Jill
    649.5'5'087

Printed and bound in China

Contents

Acknowledgements

My grateful thanks to Jill Norris who started the first special needs toy library in the UK and founded the National Association of Toy and Leisure Libraries. She inspired us all to learn so much about the value of play and toys.

I am also indebted to:

All the children who, over the years, have unwittingly supplied the material for this book.

All the parents and therapists who have shared their ideas with me for the benefit of other children. You will find their names scattered throughout the book. The royalties earned from their contributions will benefit the National Association of Toy and Leisure Libraries.

All my toy library friends and the staff at NATLL for their encouragement, suggestions and advice.

Judy Denziloe for the inspiration for the 'What to do With ...' section at the back of the book. In 'Fun and Games — Practical Leisure Ideas for People with Profound Disabilities' she includes many ideas for profitably using waste materials. I have added similar ideas relevant to children's play.

Jill Hunter for her delightful illustrations, and Stuart Wynn-Jones, Anita Jackson and Caroline Gould for supplementary pictures.

Ann Kirk for her good humoured and meticulous editing.

And particularly to my husband, John, who has acted as critic and sounding board throughout the writing of this book.

Foreword

*'We do not stop playing because we grow old,
we grow old because we stop playing.'*

Those of us who are privileged to know Roma Lear
suspect that she could have been the inspiration of
George Bernard Shaw's insightful remark. Her chirpy
smile, infectious laughter and playful soul have kept
her young beyond her years. On these pages she
unfolds for us the magic of play which modern
technology tries to capture but rarely succeeds.

For example, Roma reminds us that any object can
be transformed into an exciting plaything by the
creative talents and skilful hands of a child or adult
playmate. Expensive toys are not necessary for play;
even the most mundane of materials can be 'magically'
recreated as children's playthings.

Another magical property of play is the way it unites
peoples of all ages and cultures who share a common
heritage in the games and play activities of childhood.
In today's world, these traditions are frequently
belittled and ignored. Roma brings together ideas for
toys from her many friends around the world and from
her own and others' memories of childhood, to form
a compendium of ideas that escape the bounds of
culture and age.

Here too is the antidote to those pessimists, be they
children or adults, who are bored with play because
they have tried everything! These pages are bursting
with ideas; some of which are older than any of us and
yet presented afresh for a new generation of players.
Indeed the paradox of play is that it is often old yet
always new.

FOREWORD

Roma's special expertise has been in designing and adapting playthings for children who many think could never play; boys and girls with severe and multiple disabilities. But when all their senses are engaged and special adaptations are made to circumvent their handicaps, they too can experience the sense of achievement, as well as enjoyment, which comes through play. For them and their families, that's magic!

Above all though, play produces the miracle of laughter. This uniquely human gift is insufficiently practised in the busyness of modern living. Yet relationships are forged and friendships nurtured as we laugh and joke together. Just think what the world would be like if we adults rediscovered our childish capacity of playing and laughing together. In this book, Roma Lear offers you the elixir of youth. Taste it and discover for yourself the magic of play.

Dr Roy McConkey
Vice-President, National Association of Toy and
Leisure Libraries

Introduction

As a teacher, I was always interested in making things for my pupils. This creativity was due partly to my Froebel training, and partly to my ingenious mother who taught me to knit and sew and 'be good with my hands'. When my work took me to an orthopaedic hospital ward (long before the introduction of hospital play schemes and 'play ladies'), most of my time was taken up with school activities, but sometimes these had to go by the board. A child might be homesick and miserable, or in pain or discomfort, and much more in need of distraction than learning. Increasingly, I began to realise that my job did not finish at 3.30 pm when the teas were wheeled in. From then until bedtime and before the start of school next day were long hours, when some of the children would be bored and probably very naughty! Those over the worst stage of their treatment were desperate for something interesting to do. I began filling bags with play kits they could manage on their own or with a ward friend. Because of their treatment, some children might be lying in awkward positions, perhaps with legs on traction, one arm out of use or unable to turn their heads. By using tapes, clothes pegs, paper clips, safety pins and magnets, I learnt to invent ways of keeping pencils to hand and all else from falling off the bed.

Then I 'retired' to have our family and, like many mums with young children, became involved with a play group. At first this was held in a neighbour's house for a few children who lived in the road. Then we graduated to a much larger one for a boisterous group of under-fives. Many of the more energetic ideas in this book date from that time. Parents of today's lively pre-school children may like to try them out.

INTRODUCTION

One day, back in the 1960s, I chanced to switch on the radio as Mrs Jill Norris was describing the toy library she had recently started. She had collected toys and games specially suitable for children with disabilities. This play equipment could be borrowed for a period, then exchanged for more — just like books from the public library. We began a stimulating correspondence, and before long Kingston-upon-Thames had a toy library too! A new interest was added to my life, as I began to make and adapt toys to suit my new young friends.

In those days there were few commercial toys available for children with special needs. As time went by, manufacturers began to listen to toy librarians and, before long, we could buy chunky jigsaws with knobs on the pieces and other delights. Now there are many more specially designed toys available (at a price), and modern technology makes play possible for children who might otherwise be left out. Even so, we still have problems. Some people believe that all children with special needs should play with 'normal' toys. For many, of course, this is perfectly possible, but for others it may be a goal to aim at. A homemade toy could make a good starting point. Take a posting box for example. Most of the simple ones on sale have at least three holes to accommodate different shapes. For some children this can be totally bewildering, but if they first play with a homemade posting box with only one hole, then progress to two, in time they will understand the posting principle and be ready to make full use of the commercial version.

The number of manufactured toys available to any one child can often be limited. Parents at the toy library frequently tell me about the problems they have when they search the toy shop shelves. Maybe the child is too large — or the toy too small! That can usually be put right by buying or making a jumbo version. Perhaps the toy is too heavy, too bulky, too fragile or too complicated. Perhaps the child has a craze for cars and nothing else interests him. Perhaps, quite simply, nothing really interests him. Whatever the problem, hopefully help is at hand somewhere between the pages of this book.

The games and activities suggested need very little or no preparation. They can be enjoyed in everyday situations and only require natural objects or items found around the house — plus, on your part, a little imagination and a sense of fun. The toys are all Do It Yourself, and many can be made by anyone who can use a pair of scissors and a paint brush. Others need elementary sewing or carpentry skills.

The ideas are arranged under the headings of the five senses, and are classified as 'instant' (self explanatory!), 'quick' (can be made in an evening), or 'long-lasting' (taking a weekend or more to make).

If you have never made a toy before — and you are in good company — start with something simple (labelled 'instant' or 'quick') that you feel will be attractive and useful to your child. Read the 'Before you begin' section for instructions on toy safety, and useful tips.

Children with special needs frequently find themselves on the receiving end of other people's generosity. It may sometimes be difficult to provide opportunities for them to experience the joy of giving. There are ideas scattered through the book for things children can make as presents for each other or for an adult.

As you read on you may say to yourself 'How simple! Why didn't I think of that?', or, 'I used to do that when I was a child, but I had forgotten all about it'. This is my justification for including some elementary and traditional ideas. They can give excellent play value.

I know a nursery teacher who sometimes wakes up saying to herself 'Now what shall we do today?' She opens her copy of 'Play Helps' at random and more often than not she finds an idea to start her off. The pages that follow will not give you a play programme, but I hope they will be the start of many happy playtimes — with only a whiff of therapy! The wide margins to the pages can be used for your comments and notes.

I wish you many happy hours of creativity followed by even happier playtimes.

Introduction to the Fourth Edition

This little volume started its life in 1977, and is still known by some as 'The Orange Book'! It was followed in 1990 by 'More Play Helps' — a further collection of ideas for toys and activities for children with special needs. This time the bulk of the material was contributed by professionals and parents, who were willing to share their clever ideas with others.

'Play Helps' has already undergone two revisions. In this third one, for the fourth edition, it follows the same format as its predecessors. So what is new?

Many more toys and activities have been added to the best ideas from both 'Play Helps' and 'More Play Helps'.

For easier reference, the contents of every chapter appear at the beginning. This list replaces an index. Hopefully, it will encourage you to browse through the pages and mark on it any ideas you may come across and might like to try later.

New additions are the sections on 'Making play possible' and 'Before you begin — Hints on toy-making'. Read the former if your child has difficulty in keeping her toys to hand and, in any case, be sure to read the latter. It will help you to produce safe toys for the child in mind, and could help you avoid making common mistakes.

Since retirement, I have become a Rent-A-Gran to several local 'frail' children, who, for whatever reason, soon tire or have less than normal strength. Their toys must be small and light. I have tried to add to the few commercial toys available to them, and make their playtimes more interesting by creating special 'one-off' long-lasting toys. These have met with acclamation from the children, their parents and therapists, so I have included them in case they may be worth copying for other children with similar needs. The modern Gran is often far off retirement age, but perhaps there is a lucky child with a Great Gran or friend, who has basic sewing skills and the time to have a go.

You will find suggestions for play — indoors or out; for one child or a group; for children with minimal special needs or those who are multiply challenged, and for all those in between whose play needs may be as numerous and diverse as the children themselves.

At the back of the book, you will find hints on how to make wonderful toys that will cost you nothing!

April, 1996   Roma Lear

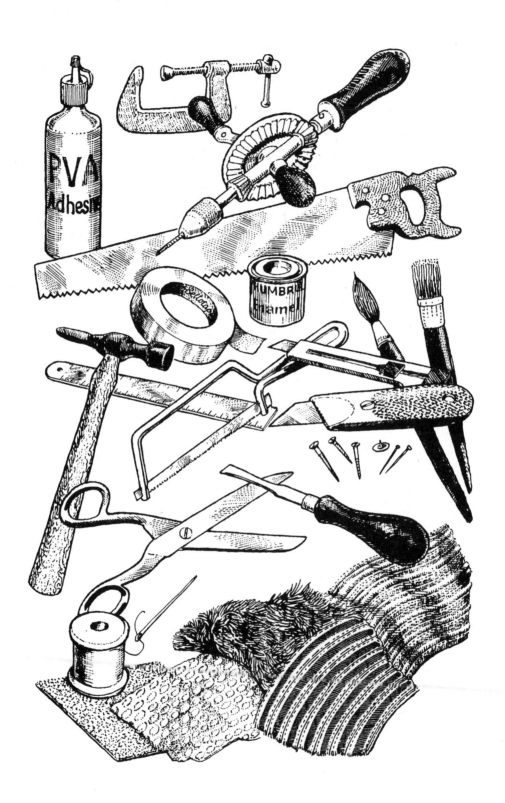

Before you begin

SOME HINTS ON TOYMAKING

The very first thing you must think about is *safety*. These days there are rigorous safety standards for manufactured toys, but even so I guess scarcely a week passes without the Casualty Department of your local hospital having to help a child in trouble through play. We all know how inquisitive children can be. Small fingers can soon stretch a little hole into a big one and innards that should be inaccessible are soon explored. They also have voracious appetites and, if small pieces of toy are not eaten, they might easily be poked in ears or noses. Please consider the safety factor extra carefully if you make feely bags or rattles, and make sure you select contents that will be harmless if they are likely to escape.

Thankfully, most children emerge from childhood unscathed and this is due to the common sense and vigilance of their carers. They know the children's habits and steer them away from trouble! When making toys for children with special needs, an even larger dose of commonsense is essential. The special cushion made for Sarah (p. 12) was stuffed with polystyrene chips — a material that should never be used with young children. But Sarah was long past the stage of putting things in her mouth, and her hands certainly did not have the strength to tear the cushion cover. Her cushion needed to be light and tactile. It was made specially for her as a 'one-off' toy, and I felt the rustling of the polystyrene chips might add to its attraction. The children around her were also passive and gentle, so there was no danger of her cushion falling into the wrong hands. The moral of this paragraph is — before you make any toy in this book consider what might happen to it! Perhaps you may need to modify the design, e.g. use lighter materials, if the toy is likely to be thrown, or make it heavier, if the child in question needs it to be made more stable.

When making a long-lasting toy always use the best materials available. The toy will look good, last longer and be a pleasure to make. Use birch plywood or Medium Density Fibreboard for wooden toys. Both sand down well, and you will avoid splinters or rough edges. New fabric is much stronger than some which has been through the wash many times. Use it double, or back it with calico for extra strength. Pay attention to seams. Stitch them twice and oversew to prevent them splitting. Sew buttons on *very* securely with strong button thread. PVA adhesive is excellent for sticking paper or card and is water-solvent if spilt. (A useful tip — if you spill some on a woollen garment, simply put it in the freezer overnight. In the morning you can pick off the brittle adhesive!) Poster paints, powder paints and felt pens sold as suitable for school use will be non-toxic. Humbrol enamel, sold in small pots for painting models, is safe for toys. It is made in lovely bright colours, covers most surfaces with only one coat and is quick drying. Polyurethane varnish is non-toxic when it is dry, and forms a good hard protective covering. Polyester fibre is sold at craft shops and upholstery departments etc. The bag should be labelled 'suitable for toy making' and marked with the CE safety mark.

The great advantage of making special toys — apart from the fun of it — is that they can be personalised for their user, and adapted to suit. Rattles and stability have already been touched upon, but perhaps a toy may need to be larger — or smaller; heavier — or lighter; made more simple — (make fewer pieces) or more difficult (increase the number). A toy can be thrown together as a five-minute wonder and soon end up in the bin, or it can be constructed with care and become a treasured possession which lasts for years. Circumstances alter cases, and the choice is yours.

All the toys in this book have been tried and tested with children, and all have proved their worth. Some have general appeal, others have been specially made to fill a particular play need, but all have been given the 'thumbs up' by the children. My less successful efforts have been discretely carried away by the dustman!

SOME MATERIALS USED

Bells	From a craft or pet shop.
Buddies or Sticky Fixers	Small plastic pads with adhesive both sides.
Button thread	Strong, twisted, waxed thread. Used for mobiles, sewing on buttons.
Diffraction paper	A magical paper with a shiny surface. Hold it in different positions to catch the light, and wonderful patterns and colours are revealed. From Edu-Play (p. 4).
Dowel	Rod of wood, pine or ramin (stronger). Made in various thicknesses. From wood yards, DIY stores.
Dycem	A plastic sheet with special non-slip qualities. Can be ordered from Boots the Chemists, medical suppliers.
Fablon	Tough, sticky-backed plastic. Used for covering tables, etc. From DIY shops.
Fish grit	Used to cover the bottoms of acquaria. Sold by the bag at pet shops.
Magnetic tape	A strip of pliable, magnetised, rubber-like plastic, with an adhesive backing. Cut to size with scissors, peel off the protective paper and apply to toys as required. From

	educational suppliers and some DIY stores.
Magnets	Those used throughout this book are the disc kind. These are easier to stick to a toy than the horseshoe type, and keep their magnetism well if you remember to replace the 'keeper' on the face of the magnet after play. From craft shops.
Masking tape	A paper tape with a special adhesive which makes it easy to remove. From stationers.
Plastic foam	Used in upholstery. From specialist shops, street markets.

List of mail-order firms

All the materials used in making the toys are available in the High Street or DIY stores, but if personal shopping is difficult here is a short list of mail-order firms.

Beckfoot Mill
Clock Mill, Denholm, Bradford, West Yorkshire
BD13 4DN
Tel: 01274 830063
    For squeakers, felt off-cuts, etc.

Craft Depot
1, Canvin Court, Somerton Business Park,
Somerton, Somerset TA11 6SB
Tel: 01458 274727
    For plastic canvas, touch'n play music buttons,
    etc.

Edu-Play
Units H and I, Vulcan Business Centre, Vulcan
Road, Leicester LE5 3EB
Tel: 01533 525827
    For diffraction paper and bells.

Escor Toys
Elliott Road, Bournemouth BH11 8JP
Tel: 01202 591081
    For a range of peg toys.

Hope Education
Orb Mill, Huddersfield Road, Oldham, Lancashire
OL4 2ST
Tel: 01616 336611
    For blank dice, scissors – various.

Just Fillings
Dept. PC, 1 Beechroyd, Pudsey, West Yorkshire
LS28 8BH
Tel: 01274 691965
    For polyester fibre.

NES Arnold
Ludlow Hill Road, West Bridgford, Nottingham
NG2 6HG
Tel: 01159 452201
    For general educational supplies, magnetic tape,
    special scissors for children.

Nottingham Rehab
Ludlow Hill Road, West Bridgford, Nottingham
NG2 6HD
Tel: 0115 945 2345
    For Dycem and special scissors for children.

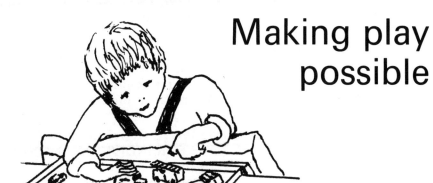

Making play possible

EVERYONE CARING FOR CHILDREN WITH SPECIAL needs knows how difficult it can often be to keep toys within reach of the child who is playing with them—and, occasionally, out of reach of the one who shouldn't be! All children who, for whatever reason, are unable to choose and fetch their own toys need help before they can start to play.

Cot and pram toys are easily bought for babies. Such toys will neither appeal nor be appropriate for older children who, because of their disabilities, still have to spend part of their time in a cot. They need their own playthings adapted for cot use. Other children are able to sit in a chair but, because of their handicap, their movements are very limited. They may have jerky, uncoordinated movements — without help their toys can be swept to the floor or knocked out of reach. What about 'frail' or sick children? They may be able to move but, in order to save them effort, their playthings need to be kept handy. Others, like the toddlers in plaster for whom the train cushion on p. 13 was specially designed, may be temporarily incapacitated. And so the list continues.

If your child has difficulty in reaching or retaining her toys, read on. Help may be among the tried and tested ideas that follow.

KEEPING TOYS WITHIN REACH

Suspending toys for children who are lying down

An Elastic Luggage Strap

Instant

This has strong hooks on both ends and can be hung across the cot so that the child can biff and grab the toys that dangle from it. It can easily be removed when the cot side needs lowering. It should be *slightly* stretched between the cot rails, so it is wise to measure before buying. Hang some toys with tape or string, but use elastic for others so that, when they are pulled and released, they will bob about.

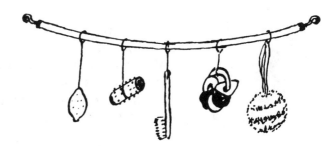

An Elastic Washing Line

Instant

Jeanette Maybanks

Here is an easy but effective way of suspending toys at any height. The brainwave came from a busy Mum who wanted to amuse her baby while he was still at the precrawling stage and floorbound on a rug. The idea could be used to hang toys within reach of any child who needs to play in a similar position. Just hang a length of elastic between two suitable points — the rungs of chairs might do. At intervals along it, attach strong bulldog clips. (These are obtainable from large stationers and office equipment suppliers.) As the name suggests, these clips grip very firmly and will withstand a fair amount of tugging. From the clips, dangle any old thing, perhaps a handkerchief, or a fluorescent sock with a rattle in the toe, a soft toy on a piece of ribbon or a glove with a little bell in a finger.

A Plastic Garden Chain

Instant
(and long lasting)

Here is another way of stringing toys in a row, either for a child in a cot, or for one lying on the floor. The chain looks attractive and, of course, is very strong — and washable! When it is firmly fixed in position, simply tie the toys to the links, position the child comfortably and let her have a go.

Goal Posts

Long-lasting

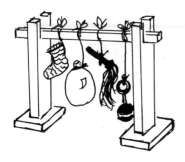

This idea is borrowed from the football pitch. A child can lie between the posts and reach all the delights that dangle from the crossbar. The posts are slotted (or fixed with brackets) into sturdy feet so that the whole frame is very stable. The crossbar rests in grooves cut in the top of the posts and, at the end of playtime, the whole contraption can be taken apart for easy storage.

All these devices should be positioned within easy reach of the children's hands so that they can biff, grab, grasp and let go as they please. Suitably placed, they may also be useful for children who can only kick.

A Hotch Potch of Toys to Biff, Grab or Pull

Instant

Select as appropriate.

- Balloons. Sausage-shaped ones are easier to hit. A few grains of rice inside, or a small bell or two, make them even more exciting.
- A bunch of ribbons or non-fray strips of material.
- Any plastic bottle with a handle, and something (safe) inside it to rattle. Fix on the lid with a dab of plastic glue, e.g. U-Hu.
- A sock with something tactile in the toe — a rattle, fir cone, squeaky toy . . . .
- A string of large buttons, perhaps with a bell (from the pet shop) added here and there.
- A plastic sweet jar with coloured cotton reels inside.
- An 'octopus' made from coloured tights stuffed with newspaper and tied together.
- A danglement made from pipe insulation tubing.
- Hang what you already have — a soft toy perhaps. Suspend it from a length of elastic, so that it will bob about if pulled and released.
- See if a plastic baby mirror appeals. This is large and shiny and has convenient holes round the edge from which to hang it.
- Thread together parts of incomplete toys, such as some stacking rings to slide over a few teething beads. Tie the ends of the threader together to form a loop.
- Hang up a bunch of rattles — much easier for a child to see and biff or grab than a single one hung up on its own.
- Thread coloured cotton reels (or till reels) on a string or as a loop.
- Use the lid from a treacle tin with a small hole punched near the rim. This lid is strong, shiny and has a well-turned edge. To make its rotations more dramatic, stick a circle of brightly-coloured Fablon on one side.
- Make a tassel from strings threaded through large buttons. Tie a knot below each button so that it stays in place and does not sink to the bottom of the string.
- Use an empty wine bag from a box of wine. Inflate it and perhaps put some adhesive stickers on it.

● Look around the kitchen for likely objects. A wooden spoon or a bunch of measuring spoons could be a winner.
● Make a strong tassel from non-fray, brightly coloured material such as lycra or sail cloth — if you have some handy!

Suggested by Christine Cousins, Judy Denziloe, Margaret Gilmore, Alison Harland, Linda Bennet School, Lilli Nielson, Fiona Priest, RNIB Advisors, Jean Vant.

See also
Bamboo Mobile, p. 110
Ship's Bell Rattle, p. 114
Octopully, p. 119
Rattle Snake, strong version, attach some hanging strings, p. 122
Grab Bags, p. 145
Amorphous Beanbag, with strings attached, p.148
Manx Feely Cushion, with strings attached, p. 148

For children playing on the floor

Instant

Pam Courtney,
Deputy Head Teacher,
St Anne's School

A child with multiple disabilities is sure to have great difficulty in keeping his toys within reach. He may have limited or uncontrolled movements, perhaps combined with poor sight or hearing. It is not surprising that a child with all these problems will soon lose interest in his play. If he pushes his toys away with an involuntary movement, there they will stay — out of reach — out of sight — and probably out of mind. The child is left with nothing to do until someone notices his plight.

Pam has suggested two simple ways to overcome this problem:

1. Playing on a Sloping Surface

If the child is playing on the floor and lying on one side, a sheet of hardboard can be placed between him and the wall. The far edge of the hardboard is raised (prop it up on the telephone directory!) so that when toys are pushed away they will slide down and back to him.

2. Playing in a Baby Bath

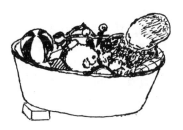

For a *small* child who is able to sit up, a baby bath with one end slightly raised makes a good 'child and toy container'. The high sides of the bath also help to keep toys to hand. Pam has found that, for some children, it is better to put plenty of toys in the bath — not just one or two. This bonanza cannot be ignored and should tempt the child to investigate — and play. As an alternative to a baby bath, you might use a plastic laundry basket. This has the added advantage that toys can be strung across it or tied to the sides — useful if the child might otherwise end up sitting on them.

For ways of keeping toys to hand for older children playing on the floor, search through the section on bed play below. The problems can be similar.

For children in bed

A Play Cushion

Quick

Susan Harvey and
Ann Hales-Tooke

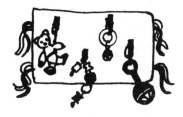

In the early days of play in hospital, these pioneering play specialists devised unusual cushions for very young patients who needed nursing in oxygen tents. In this situation the children continually lost their toys among the folds of the tent. To overcome the problem, hospital pillows, already encased in washable plastic, were given attractive, removable outer covers. Rings or loops were firmly attached to one side, and tie strings to the other. Rattles, soft toys, etc. were attached to the loops as needed, and the tie strings fixed the cushions securely to the cot bars — to avoid any danger of them falling onto the children.

Method
- Use *new* material. It is stronger. Make sure it is washable.
- Choose a plain colour. The toys show up better.
- Keep the strings attached to the toys fairly short to avoid tangling.
- Remember to hold the child's interest by changing the toys now and then.

A Special Play Cushion for Sarah

Long-lasting

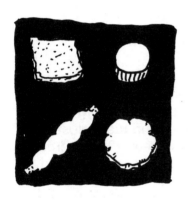

Imagine Sarah and her problems. She was seventeen, and severely handicapped. Although able to see, she showed no interest in looking at anything. She could hear, but not speak, and seemed quite unmoved by music or any other sounds. She had hardly any movement in her limbs and her days were spent for the most part in her special chair. Unless frequently coaxed to hold something, her beautiful, elegant and unused hands lay resting on her lap.

In an effort to please her, I thought of making a one-off lap cushion. By chance, that morning I received a letter from Mme Schneider (whose toys are included elsewhere in this book). She told me about the toys she made for visually impaired children. To get maximum colour contrast she used black and white. Perhaps I could attract Sarah's attention by using high contrast colours. What about a pleasant feel, nice smell, and a chance to make a noise?

A raid on the 'bits' bag produced some black satin and some fur fabric — also black. The satin was chosen for the top of the cushion, and the four attachments which provided the play element were sewn to it. One was made from a circle of startlingly white material, gathered round the edge like a mob cap, and filled with little bells. Another was a 'shocking pink' tube of stretch velvet, stuffed with marbles. It was attached to the cushion at both ends, like a handle. The marbles could be squeezed up and down the tube. The third attachment was made from brilliant green material and was shaped like a tree stump. It was filled with fish grit (cheap, and easy to buy from the pet shop). It gave a pleasing, squelchy sensation when pinched. The last was a square cushion, brilliant yellow in colour, and stuffed with lavender (like a peculiar piece of ravioli!). It was attached to the cushion only at the centre of its base so that it fitted into the hand and was easy to crunch — so releasing the smell. The fur fabric was used for the bottom of the cushion which was then stuffed with polystyrene chips. The hope was that these would make a rustling sound if ever Sarah moved her hands. The fur fabric resting on her knees was intended to give her a warm, comfortable sensation, like nursing a friendly cat. Was it a success?

How difficult to say! Certainly Sarah's hands could sometimes be seen moving voluntarily over her cushion, and on entering the room in the morning she seemed happier when her cushion was on her knee. An act of faith perhaps, but I think she responded to my efforts.

Note
Polystyrene chips were suitable in this situation, but should **not** be used for toys. They are dangerous if swallowed.

A Train Cushion

Long-lasting

Designed by
Jean Gregg
and made by
Sarah Bondoux,
Play Specialists

This delightful play cushion was designed to meet the particular needs of small children on abduction frames in a hospital ward. Their legs and hips were immobilised, but their hands were free to play with anything they could reach. This large cushion acted as a toy holder. It was stuffed with an oblong of thick plastic foam. This made it rigid enough to stand unsupported at the side of the cot and was long enough to form a cosy play corner, hiding the child from the rest of the ward. The play leaders thought this was an important point. Children love to creep into a hidey-hole now and then, to 'get away from it all'. The train cushion, wedged between the cot bars and the mattress, gave the illusion of privacy and helped to fill this need.

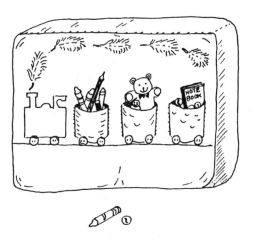

The children found the appliqued picture on the cover very attractive. Across the middle chugged an engine towing three carriages. The 'steam' from the funnel was represented by a strip of swansdown which flowed up and along the top of the cushion. Of course it was stitched securely along its entire length. (Not everyone has swansdowns in their 'bits' bag! Ric-rac braid could make a poor substitute.) The three brightly coloured felt carriages formed pockets in which small toys, finger puppets, crayons, etc. could be stored. The lucky child having her turn with the cushion could help herself to whatever she wanted.

As well as making play possible for bed-bound children, the cushion can be propped up against a wall or used flat on the floor. When not being used for play, it makes a very attractive nursery picture.

A Play Table for Bed or Floor

Quick

Alison Wisbeach,
Occupational Therapist

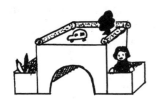

Children in hospital are provided with special tables to fit over their beds. For the child who is nursed at home Alison has thought up a quickly-made play table. She begins with a *sturdy* cardboard box, (e.g. one from the Off Licence) and cuts a knee hole in one side. Plastic foam pipe wrap is glued to the top edges of the other three sides, making a retaining wall to prevent toys from falling off. Finally, she glues empty shoe boxes to each side to hold toys, felt pens, paper, etc. Thus equipped the child should have everything to hand for a happy play time.

A Revolving Play Tidy

Long-lasting

Karen Padgett Chandler,
Hospital Play Specialist

Think of a cake icing turntable with containers of different sizes fixed to it and you will understand the principle behind this useful play tidy.

The original model was designed to make play easier for a group of four children sharing activities at a drawing table while waiting their turn at a Hospital Out-Patients' Department. The containers held paper, pencils, felt pens, sticky shapes, scissors, etc. The revolving top of the turntable made sure these were *within reach* of everyone.

It is this last feature which can make a revolving play tidy a boon to a child with short arms or very little mobility.

14

The play tidy consists of two parts: a circular rotating top cut from plywood, attached by a long screw to a firm wooden base. This has non-slip rubber feet or Dycem (p. 3) attached to the bottom to prevent it slipping.

Various plastic boxes, tins with safe rounded edges, a plastic sink tidy, etc. are screwed to the revolving top. For easy access, the tall containers are put in the centre and the shallow ones arranged around the edge.

To make it easy to turn, the top should overlap the base. It is also a good idea to make the base fairly thick. This will raise the revolving part well clear of the tabletop to avoid any possible danger of small fingers being squashed in between.

For a less robust turntable tidy, use a plastic cake-icing turntable and attach the containers to the top with Blu-tac or a double-sided fixer like 'Buddies' or 'Sticky Fixers'.

A Reacher

Quick

Alison Wisbeach,
Occupational Therapist

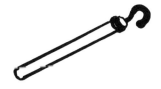

Some of us are familiar with the reachers available commercially for adults. (By squeezing a handle at one end of a rod, a claw at the other can be made to pick up dropped objects.) Smaller versions are available for children, but not all can manage the controlled movements they require. Alison has come to the rescue again! She suggests a simple reacher made from a length of dowel with a large cup hook screwed in one end. With this cheap and handy little device, straying toys can be hooked back into play.

Of course, the length and thickness (and consequently the weight) of the dowel can be adjusted to suit the user. Just drill a small hole in one end of the dowel, screw in the cup hook, and bind round the end with button thread or thin string to stop it from splitting.

For children in wheelchairs

A Three-sided Clothes Horse

Quick

Leicester Toy Library

One day a tiny little girl visited the Leicester Toy Library. She was in an extra small wheelchair. Her Mum was looking for suitable toys that she could watch and perhaps reach out and touch. An ingenious member of the toy library staff came up with the perfect idea — hang toys from a doll's clothes horse from a laundry play set! This was just the right size to fit snugly round the wheelchair and could be tied to the arms to make it stable. All sorts of toys could be hung from the rails. The cage and bells from a roller rattle was fixed to the top one. This turned out to be a stroke of genius, for everyone passing by was tempted to give the cage a whirl — much to the delight of the little girl. Toys like pull-string music boxes, rattles, and paper toys that moved in the draught were hung from other rails. Using this simple, ready-made frame, the child was surrounded on three sides by attractive playthings, easily changed when they no longer appealed. Safe and cosy behind her toy frame, she could still watch everything that was going on around her.

The Whirly Line

Instant

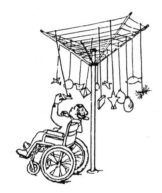

A Tabletop Necklace

Quick

Mrs Crane,
Teacher,
The Manor School

When the warm weather is here and the washing is out of the way, why not use the whirly line as an out door toy holder? The fact that it revolves adds to its attraction, and a determined child can tug his way to the toy of his choice.

For children playing at a table

Tying toys to a necklace for a *child* to wear is obviously not a good idea, because of the risk of it tightening round his neck. But to make a string of playthings which can be looped over a tabletop is a safe way of keeping toys within reach.

The first tabletop necklace I came across was made — in desperation — by a teacher in a school for children with severe learning difficulties. In her group were several lively lads, and one who was not able to move from his wheelchair. This boy was quiet and gentle. His favourite occupation was to shake and rattle plastic toys. Unfortunately, his class mates often took a fancy to his playthings and grabbed them from him, leaving him very upset. (Naturally!) His teacher came up with this answer. She collected all his favourite toys and tied each to the middle of a strip of nylon tape (scrap from a factory). She cut three more pieces of the same tape, each three times the width of the play table. She plaited these together and, at intervals, both ends of the tape with a toy attached were incorporated into the plait.

This long 'necklace' was laid across the tabletop and passed under it so that the ends could be knotted together to make a loop. The boy could now sit at the table and pull the necklace towards him until he reached the toy of his choice. He might go for 'Flip Fingers', a large plastic ring with strings of buttons attached, a plastic car, a pair of plastic scissors, a trainer ball with holes in it and a bell inside, a string of large beads, a bunch of keys or various rattles. At last he could enjoy his favourite activity in uninterrupted peace.

A Tabletop Play Corner

Quick

Judy Denziloe,
Project Coordinator,
Planet

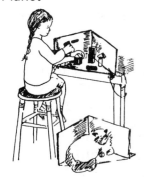

How can you help a seated child keep her toys conveniently on the top of the table when her jerky movements often sweep them to the floor? All you need is a sizeable square cardboard carton from the supermarket. Cut it diagonally in half and use one piece to make the triangular play space. Toys can be played with on the floor of the box and the high sides will prevent them from being pushed away. If appropriate, you can make holes in the sides and dangle toys from them. The tabletop play corner is certain to need stabilising. Perhaps sticking it to the table with masking tape or Blu-tac will be sufficient. Otherwise, try wedging it in place with something heavy — the telephone directory? sandbags? a covered brick? — or make a few holes in the bottom of the sides and tie the whole affair down securely.

A Play Box

Quick

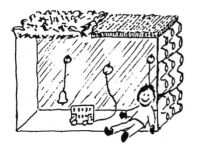

For a child with a visual impairment, this useful device serves two purposes. It keeps toys within reach and the textured outside encourages small fingers to explore the shape, giving the child an idea of the size of the play area.

Stick some interesting textures to the outside of the box. For ideas, turn to p. 151. Make holes in the sides here and there and fix loops of elastic to them. Double the elastic in half, tie a knot to form the loop, then poke the two ends through the hole. Tie a *large* knot — that will not pull through — on the outside of the box. Tie toys to the loops. The floor of the box makes a useful surface for building games, because the bricks cannot topple out of reach.

For children playing in the car

A Play Pinny

Quick

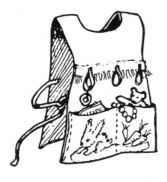

Over the years our toy library at Kingston-upon-Thames has been supplying pinnies of an appropriate size to children with visual or physical problems. With the help of this useful little cover-up, toys attached to the loops cannot be dropped or pushed out of reach. On a long journey, a play pinny can be a boon to any small child strapped in his safety seat, possibly with no-one beside him to retrieve dropped playthings. The pinny ensures that child and toys stay together!

The basic pattern is just an oblong of material, the width of the child's shoulders, with a hole cut in the middle for his head to go through. A pocket is made along the bottom of the front. It is divided down the middle with a row of stitching to make a separate pocket for each hand. Three loops of tape are sewn to the front of the pinny. It is wise to stitch a reinforcing strip behind these, and attach them very securely. They will have to withstand a considerable amount of pulling and tweaking. The raw edges are neatened by binding round the neck and hemming the top of the pocket, sides and bottom of the back. Short lengths of tape are stitched to each side. When these are tied together, they stop the pinny from rucking up when worn. Now all that is needed are some little surprises to hide in the pockets, (crunchy paper, a fir cone?) and some suitable toys to tie to the loops of tape (rattle, teether, soft toy?).

For children who tend to scatter their toys

A Picture Frame

Instant

Jenny Buckle,
Play Leader and Parent

It is so easy for Lego bricks, Play People with all their accessories—or any other toy with lots of small pieces—to be scattered over the tabletop, but put them inside a picture frame and the problem is solved!

This idea is particularly useful for older children with limited reach.

Magnetic Tape and a Metal Playboard

Quick

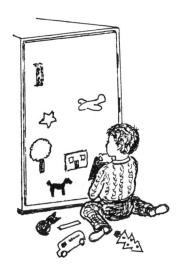

This method is fun for all children, but it is particularly *useful* for those with a visual handicap or poor hand-eye coordination. Play pieces with the magnetic tape applied will stick to the board until the child chooses to move them. It is even possible to make the adhesion light or firm, according to the amount of magnetic tape that is applied.

Magnetic tape can always be obtained from Educational Suppliers (p. 4) and can sometimes be found in High Street shops. It is sold by length and comes in ribbon form with a self-adhesive backing. Cut off the required length and stick it to the underside of small toys, mosaic shapes for pattern making, 'push together puzzles' (p. 88), small containers, or what you will.

Provide a metal playboard from a toy shop, usually sold complete with letters, numbers and shapes. A large, shallow biscuit-baking tray works just as well, but this is lighter and will probably need anchoring down.

SOME WAYS OF ADAPTING TOOLS AND TOYS FOR INDIVIDUAL NEEDS

Handles

1. *Too short*
   - For sand pit or gardening tools, search at the garden centre for lightweight tools (intended for elderly or disabled gardeners). These tools have an extending attachment that can be fitted to the handles.
   - For pencils, saw off a suitable length of bamboo garden cane and wedge the pencil inside the hollow centre.
   - Paint brushes with long handles are obtainable at good toy shops or Educational Suppliers (p. 4).

2. *Too long*
   - Cut them down, or find a smaller equivalent, e.g. make-up brushes can be used for painting. Bridge or diary pencils are short and thin.

3. *Too narrow*
- Pad them out with layers of rubber bands.
- Bandage tightly with strips of rag.
- Wind round with plastic foam and tie firmly.
- Poke a paint brush or pencil through the holes in a plastic golf practise ball.
- Use bicycle handle bar grips.
- Consult your therapist and buy specially shaped handles from a medical supplier.

Inset Puzzles: Alternative Ways of Removing and Replacing the Pieces

Most manufacturers now offer a range of inset tray puzzles with knobs attached to individual pieces. These make them more manageable for some children, but however hard the toy industry tries to help, it cannot be expected to meet the special needs of everyone. Often a small adaptation to a commercial puzzle will turn a session of frustration into one of achievement. Here are four alternatives to knobs.

1. *Raise up the inserted piece*
Cut out an identical shape in plywood, or thick card, and stick it to the bottom of the original piece. This will now stand proud of the tray and can be handled by grasping it round the edge.

2. *Screw a plasticised cup hook into the inset piece*
If this protrudes through to the underside, file it flat and smooth. This idea dates from the early days of toy libraries when Audrey Stevenson, an eminent and ingenious toy designer, found that by using this simple device some children with severe hand-function problems could manage to hook out the pieces and replace them correctly. Being slender, the cup hooks hardly obscure the picture — as can happen when large knobs are attached.

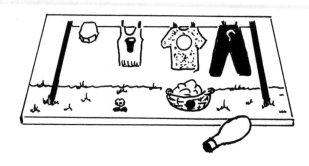

3. *Use a plastic golf tee*
This makes a fairly unobtrusive knob. It can be just the right shape for a child with small hands to grasp easily. Drill right through the inset piece and countersink a small depression on the underside. Poke the tee through the hole so that the tip protrudes. Rub this with a hot metal object to melt the plastic and make it fill up the hole. For this operation you can use the back of an old spoon. When heating it up, wrap a cloth round the handle, for this will also get hot. **Take care!** When the plastic is cold, the tee will be fused firmly in place.

4. *Use drawing pins and a magnet*
This idea has a strong appeal for children. They seem to see it as some kind of magic! It is really very simple. A steel drawing pin is pushed into the inset piece and a strong round magnet is glued to a handle. (Use a firm adhesive like Araldite or Evostick.) Place the magnet on the pin and — Hey Presto! — out comes the inset piece! For children who cannot hold a handle, the magnet can be sewn to a fabric strap with a Velcro fastening. The strap can be worn as a bracelet, or over the child's hand — like a benign knuckle duster! *Remember to remove the drawing pins after the play session if there is any chance of them endangering other children.*

Suggested by Jenny Buckle, The Disabled Living Foundation, Alison Wisbeach and R.L.

STABILISING TOYS

A Quick Fix for Light Toys and Paper

1. *A loop of masking tape*
Make a loose ring of tape round your finger, sticky side out. Slide it off your finger. Squash the loop flat, and it will make a double-sided fixer.

2. *Double-sided Sellotape*
More expensive than (1) above, but it can be applied as a strip.

3. *Other commercial fixers* like Blu-tack, Sticky Fixers, etc.

4. *Bulldog clips, clothes pegs or large paper fasteners* — the curved wire kind.
These will keep paper on a clip board from rucking up.

More Durable Fixers for Larger and Heavier Items

1. *Dycem*
This is a rubber-like material. It ensures that items — like the biscuit-baking tray mentioned on p. 19 — will stick firmly to the table. It is sold for stabilising plates, mixing bowls, etc., and is available from some of the suppliers on p. 4.

2. *Plastic suckers*
Some toys for babies are already mounted this way. For good adhesion and to stop the toy from rocking, it may be necessary to use several together, or you could try a soap saver which already has a group of suckers both sides.

3. *A G cramp*
This is a very secure way of anchoring a board game or toy with a flat base to a tabletop. A toy such as a garage or a dolls' house may need mounting on a bigger base of plywood or hardboard to give the G cramp a surface to grip.

4. *A covered brick (or therapy sandbag)*
This is useful for weighting something down, e.g. a box full of small pieces — (put the brick inside the box), or for making a temporary retaining wall round a play space. Cover the brick with fabric to make it look and feel more attractive.

P.S. Don't forget the really simple ways of keeping toys in place. Velcro, string, elastic, tape, or the telephone directory will often do the trick!

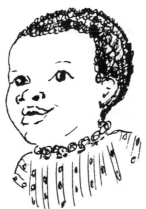

Making the most of SIGHT

THE IMPORTANCE OF LEARNING TO LOOK

All children need to be encouraged to use their eyes and think about what they see. For those who find it difficult to concentrate, or those who appear to take little interest in their environment, a special effort must be made to try to provide them with things they will really *want* to look at. A new toy can often help, especially if it combines colour, movement and sound ... so, too, can a looking game. There are some of both in this chapter.

As well as interesting things to look at, children also need *time*. Time to look and discover at their own pace, and time from us for encouragement and guidance.

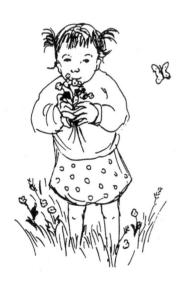

Apart from the pleasurable and educational advantages a 'good look' can bring, for some children it is an essential skill that must be well learnt. Imagine yourself in the shoes of a profoundly deaf child. You cannot hear people calling to you, so you must learn to watch for signs that they want to communicate. You cannot hear the lorry coming, so you must learn to look extra carefully before you cross the road. Slow-learners, too, often need much encouragement to use their eyes, so that they can take in what they see. Some children may stare, but seldom really *look*. Others flutter like a butterfly from one object to the next without really noticing anything properly. Without our help, all the information their eyes can give them may make little impression. Perhaps a child is playing on the grass and picks a bunch of daisies. Gathering them may have been fun, but then she just throws them down. That could be the end of that! But if she can be persuaded to carry them home, arrange them in an egg cup and put them in the middle of the table for all the family to admire, she will have been given several chances to have a good look at them. During the course of a busy day, it is so easy to let opportunities like the daisy-gathering incident pass by. This chapter will suggest many other 'instant' ways of helping a child learn to look with advantage. They can be found at the beginning of each section, followed by toys to make and, finally, games to play.

Note

When you are making or buying toys for the enjoyment of a child with a visual impairment, follow the 'BBC' code suggested by the RNIB, for this can help him to make the most of his sight. The initials stand for **B**ig, **B**right and **C**olourful.

Big. Big toys are obviously easier for your child to see, and therefore to find. Older children might use a magnification aid to make the smaller toys they enjoy more visible.

Bright. This means presenting toys and play material in the best possible light, perhaps arranging a play area near a window. For some children an angle-poise lamp may be helpful. Consult your therapist.

Colourful. Choose toys with strong colours, and make sure they do not merge into the background. Putting a cot sheet over a heavily patterned carpet can often solve this problem.

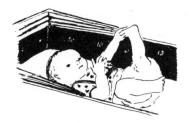

MOBILES

Perhaps little cave babies lying on their sabre-toothed tiger rugs at the beginning of history gurgled happily as they watched the leaves flutter in the breeze and the fluffy white clouds drift across the mouth of the cave. The modern baby lying in his cot or pram, more often than not, may have only the blank ceiling to look at. This situation can sometimes be part of the daily lives of older children too. Unable to move independently, sick, or injured and in plaster, they have to stay where they are put. Under any of these circumstances, a colourful and interesting mobile can soothe, intrigue and certainly help to relieve boredom.

There are mobiles of every description in the shops. Delightful as they may be, they can have their limitations. Some may be too small or too complicated for the children to see easily, and all are fairly costly. To hold a child's interest, a mobile should be changed quite often, and this could make a hole in the budget. How much more satisfactory to enlist the help of the family and make one to fit your own requirements.

General advice

Before the action begins, have a quiet think. How big do you want your mobile to be? Where will you hang it? How will you suspend the rotating vanes or shapes? Will you be content with a single shape, or will you go for the more visually exciting cluster? What materials will you use?

Size
This depends on the size of the room and, to some extent, on the reason for making the mobile in the first place. Is it for domestic use or do you intend it as an arresting feature in a schoolroom?

Location
Think about the motive power. A mobile needs some movement in the air to set it going, so try to hang it in a draught, perhaps near an open window or by a radiator. Small, light mobiles can be hung almost anywhere, e.g. from a string stretched across a corner of the room. The string can be tied between two cup hooks screwed into the picture rail. A large mobile must be hung from the rafters or from a ceiling hook capable of supporting the weight.

Hanging the shapes
The following ways are commonly used:
● *A wooden coathanger.* Paint it white. Drill a few holes in it — or cut some notches in the top — to prevent the strings from bunching together or slipping off.
● *A wire coathanger.* Keep the strings in place with Sellotape.

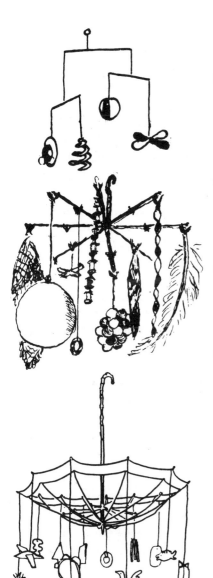

● *Short lengths of wire*. Use these to make a balanced mobile in the traditional manner. Start by hanging the bottom pair of shapes first and work upwards. This way it is easier to adjust the balance as you go. When each arm of the mobile is hanging level and rotating nicely without touching its neighbour, fix the strings in place with a dab of adhesive.

● *Intersecting thin garden canes*, say 30 cm (12″) long. Bind them together firmly in the centre where they cross. Hang shapes from the ends of the canes and from the centre. Fiddle around with them until they balance properly, then fix them in place with a dab of adhesive.

● *A plastic hoop*. This is ideal for larger mobiles. Hang it by three strings attached to the hoop at equal distances apart. When the hoop is hanging level, knot the strings together and use one for the final hanging.

● *A drip-dry carousel*. This hangs from a central hook and has plastic spokes with clothes pegs already attached. It should have no balance problems but, if it tilts, rearrange the hanging items — or add more to the higher side.

● *An old umbrella*. For hospital wards, schoolrooms and other large areas, mobiles can be hung very effectively from an old umbrella. Remove the tatty cover, but leave about 5 cm (2″) to make a strip round the edge. When the umbrella is opened, this will stop the ribs from flopping about. (The first time I made a mobile this way, I removed all the cover, and then had the tiresome job of fixing spacing strings between the ribs.) The strip of cloth can be decorated with tinsel, crêpe paper, etc. Hang the umbrella upside down and attach the mobile shapes to the ribs.

Materials

This is the creative part. Because mobiles are intended to be watched and **not touched**, almost any light and colourful material can be used. Paper of all kinds, sequins, feathers, felt, flimsy fabric, ping-pong balls, faulty compact discs — all can come in handy. Add something that will rustle, like tissue paper streamers or a string of foil milk bottle tops, and the mobile will be even more attractive to its young viewer.

What to hang on your mobile

Use cylindrical or conical shapes sparingly, they will not turn — only sway about.

Flat shapes always rotate well. If you want to be slightly more adventurous, try cutting out the shape twice, making a slit in one from the top to the middle, and in the other from the bottom to the middle. Slot the shapes together at right angles. Hang from the shape with the slot in the top.

Hang the shapes with button thread. This is a strong waxy thread with a twist in it. The twist helps the shapes to wind and unwind.

If a mobile has a theme, it is easier to think of suitable shapes to make for it. Take the weather for example. A mobile on this theme could include: the sun, clouds (fluffy white or menacing grey), strings of raindrops, a dramatic zigzag of thunder (diffraction paper?), a bunch of flimsy white net to represent fog, snowflakes cut from a paper doily (possibly stiffened with a squirt of spray starch if they tend to flop) — and so on. Perhaps a mobile to celebrate a birthday — or any other festival — would be fun to make. When inspiration flags how about trying one of the ideas that follow?

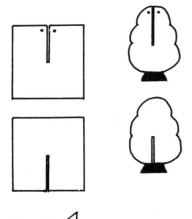

Treasures from a Country Walk

Instant

Imagine you have found a conker with its spiny shell, some acorns still attached to their cups, a large feather and a cluster of fluffy old man's beard seeds. String them up to a twig, hang it that so that it balances, and you have a beautiful mobile to remind you of the walk. Of course, it will have a limited life, but this is a point in its favour. Its viewers will not have time to grow so bored with it that they stop looking.

A Flock of Birds

These attractive little birds hang in the corner of the room where the nursery children take their daily rest.

Quick

Bedelsford School

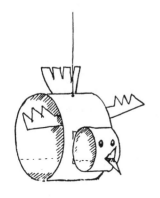

They are made entirely of white paper with only their orange beaks and black eyes to add a touch of colour. The effect is gentle and soothing — just right for rest time.

The body of each bird is made from a ring of paper (like a napkin ring), and the head is formed from a smaller one. Stick these together. Make a beak out of a diamond-shaped scrap of paper. Colour it. Fold it in half and stick it to the head. Mark in the eyes with black felt pen. If you want wings, cut both out together and stick them to the inside of the body ring. (The birds at Bedelsford School are wingless and look quite convincing.) Attach an upward-sweeping tail to give the bird a perky look — a drooping tail makes it look depressed!

A Shoal of Paper Fish

Quick

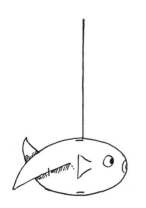

These fish have a chubby, three-dimensional look and are easy to make. Cut out two identical oval-shaped pieces of stiff paper. Decorate them while they are still flat. You might like to make each side different — some fish are like that! One side could be coloured and the other covered with diffraction paper (p. 3). This gives a striking effect when each fish is finally revolving gently on the end of its string. In each fish shape, cut a horizontal slit from the tail end to about the middle of the body. Take the two parts of the tail and overlap them so that the points stick out beyond the body. Stick or staple them together. The body now bows outwards a little. This slightly domed shape will give the fish its final 3D effect. If you want top or bottom fins, add them now. Next, stick or staple the two halves of the fish together. If it tends to collapse on you at this stage, stuff it with a scrunched-up tissue to pad it out. Add the side fins. Finally, to find the best position for the hanging thread, poke a needle through the body at the place where you think it should go, and see how the fish balances. If it doesn't, try again, but remember all the fish do not have to swim straight. The mobile looks more interesting if a few with independent spirits head for the surface of the water, and others for the sandy bottom.

Another Shoal of Fish — Felt This Time

Fairly Quick

It must be admitted that this mobile will take a little longer to make than the previous one, but it is more robust and makes a pretty present that can safely be sent through the post. Make the fish in different shapes and colours, and decorate them with sequins. First make paper patterns. If you need inspiration, look in fishy books or study the real thing at your local pet shop. Using the patterns, cut out each fish twice in felt. Sew on felt eyes and attach the sequins. It is easier to finish off properly at the back if you do this before the two halves are joined together. I like to incorporate the hanging thread in the top seam as I join the sides together. (Stab stitch, buttonhole or oversew.) To make sure it will not pull out, I tie one end of the thread round a scrap of felt, and bury it in the body of the fish. As I sew round the top of the fish, I make several extra stitches round the thread — for safety — and before I completely join the sides together, I slip in a small amount of polyester fibre to give the fish a chubbier shape.

A Mobile Within a Mobile

Quick

Susie Mason,
Toy Librarian

Susie has a delightfully simple way of making a mobile where the centre part moves independently from the outside. She starts with a round cheese box and removes the centre, leaving the rim to make a frame. This is painted in a bright colour. From the cardboard middle she cuts a shape — a face, animal, boat, flower or Christmas tree — the possibilities are endless! This shape is coloured on both sides and suspended in the centre of the frame. When both parts are hung up, each can rotate independently of the other.

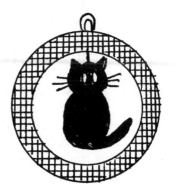

Cutting out a Single Large Shape and Decorating it

Quick

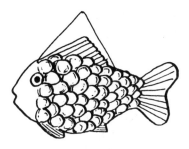

Take a piece of cardboard and cut out a familiar shape such as a car, a house or a fish. As the shape will rotate in the draught, each side could be decorated differently. Finding the right suspension point for a large mobile can present problems. Nobody wants to look at a house with subsidence or a car for ever going uphill. The solution is to hang the shape from a thread attached at two points, like a picture cord. Tie the suspending thread to these and the shape can be see-sawed like a picture on a nail, until it is hanging correctly.

A Power-driven Mobile

Long-Lasting

Have you ever poked a rubber band through both a cotton reel and a chunk of candle, anchoring it at each end with a matchstick, wound it up, then watched it crawl across the carpet? If you have, you will understand the simple mechanism which keeps this restful mobile turning for a surprisingly long time.

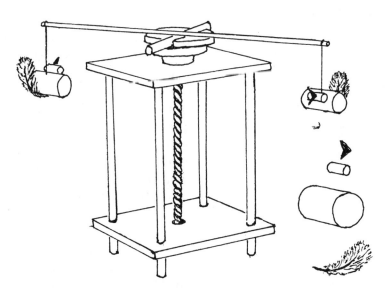

If you have elementary carpentry skill, a fretsaw, a drill and some sandpaper here is one way to make a power-driven mobile.

Materials
- Scraps of plywood
- Thin dowel
- A strong rubber band (dropped by the postman?)
- A small piece of candle
- A drinking straw
- Paper and trimmings for the two tiny birds
- A dab of glue and a scrap of Sellotape

Method
Cut two squares of plywood, say 10 × 10 cm (4″). Drill four holes in each corner of the base (to accommodate the dowel), and four more in the underside of the top. Drill through the centre of each square to make holes for the rubber band. Cut four lengths of dowel for the side supports and glue them in place. Cut two short lengths of dowel, one to anchor the band at the top and the other to act as a key to wind it up. The key needs to be small enough to fit between the supports so that it can be turned easily. Cut two circles of plywood, say 7 cm (2$\frac{3}{4}$″) diameter. Drill a hole in the centre of one and cut the other in half. (See exploded illustration.) Make a hole in the piece of candle. The easiest way of doing this without the risk of splitting it is to put a needle in a cork, heat the needle and melt out a hole just large enough to take the rubber band.

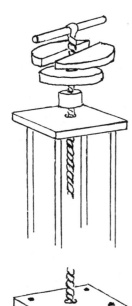

Thread the rubber band up through the base, and anchor it with the 'key' dowel. Then thread it through the top square, the candle and the bottom disc. Hold it there with the other short dowel. Glue the half circles to the bottom disc, each side of the dowel. Allow a clearance. This will make it easier to replace the band when the need arises. Fix a drinking straw across the top with Sellotape.

The Birds
These are made from two strips of paper, as for the bird mobile on p. 30. Add a scrap of coloured feather for a tail. Alternatively, hang tiny fish, Christmas baubles, paper children riding on pipe-cleaner swings — or what you will.

Turn the 'key' to wind up the band. When it is crinkly,

stand back and enjoy the result. Children find this silent and gently rotating mobile rivetting—and adults go for it in a big way!

See also
Dancing Danglement, p. 110
Bamboo Mobile, p. 110
Circular Mobile, p. 112
Convection Snake, p. 185
Button up a Mobile, p. 193

BUBBLES

Blowing bubbles is one of the sure-fire play successes of early childhood. They are mostly blown for the sheer pleasure of it but, if justification is needed for this indulgence, it can be said that watching bubbles makes a perfect 'tracking' activity. They float *slowly* in the direction of the air current and are full of entrancing colours. There is always the fun of trying to blow a huge one that will drift further than all the others before it ends in an unpredictable 'pop'. On a less aesthetic level, they are often used for teaching breath control.

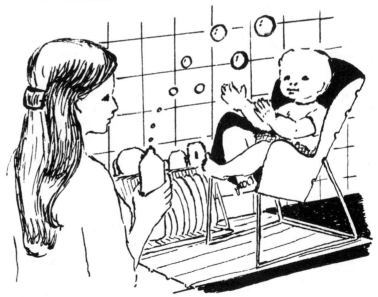

More Spectacular Bubbles and What to Do with Them

1. *Blowing a mound of bubbles*

Some children will have already discovered how do to this when they have vigorously blown through a straw into their beaker of milk — and probably been scolded for their bad manners!

Sometimes the art of 'bubbling' has to be learnt. When a straw is placed in her mouth, a child may think she is being offered a pleasant drink, and will suck instead of blow. What an unpleasant shock to end up with a mouthful of soapy water! One way to make sure this does not happen is to use a transparent drinking straw or, better still, a length of thin polythene tubing used in wine making. This can quickly be removed from the child's mouth if the liquid is seen to travel upwards.

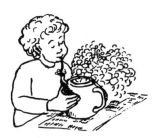

Once having learnt to bubble efficiently, the obvious place for all this frothy activity is in the bath. At other times, a lot of mess can be avoided by putting the basin of bubble mixture inside a washing-up bowl or on a tray covered with a towel. This way the bubbles can pile up and spill over the edge of the basin, but the child and her surroundings should remain dry.

When the excitement of blowing bubbles in a basin begins to pall, try using an unusual container. A teacher at the Sense Centre (for deaf/blind children) puts bubble mixture in a teapot. Try it! How about covering the basin with a colander and watching the bubbles appear through the holes or see what happens if you cover the basin with wide mesh curtaining?

Another use for a pile of bubbles is to turn them into a pattern. In the nursery class at a local school, I watched the teacher add a small amount of powder paint to the bubble mixture in a pudding basin. A little group of children raised an impressive pile of tinted bubbles. A sheet of paper was pressed gently on the top until some bubbles stuck to it. The paper was carefully lifted off and put aside to dry. We all watched the bubbles gradually pop, leaving behind a delicate pattern of overlapping circles.

2. *How to blow bubbles a different way*
One bath night my children discovered that a cotton reel (floating around as a bath toy!) made a good bubble pipe. A bubble could be blown by rubbing one end over the soap until a membrane formed, and directing a gentle stream of breath through the other. The cotton reel works just as well with bubble mixture, but it is wise to point the reel downwards to avoid the detergent trickling down the hole into the child's mouth.

3. *Blowing enormous bubbles*
At an Exploratorium (a hands-on science museum) I saw two children make a huge bubble this way. They had a metal ring, about 60 cm (2 ft) in diameter, with handles welded to each side. They dipped the hoop in a tray of bubble mixture, then ran with it. A huge sausage-shaped bubble streamed out from the hoop, growing longer and longer until it popped.

4. *The ultimate in bubble blowing*
I guess you have marvelled at a ship-in-a-bottle, but how about a child-in-a-bubble? Two hospital play specialists demonstrated how this could be done. They spread bubble mixture over the bottom of a large tray, made a loop of string — large enough to encircle a child — and attached four string handles at equal distances apart. Standing one each side of the tray, they dipped the string in the bubble mixture, lifted it carefully by the handles, (keeping the soapy membrane intact), raised it high above the child and smartly lowered it, trapping him inside the bubble.

Ideas contributed by Stephanie Clements, Pam Courtney, Christine Cousins and R.L.

An Elegant Bubble-blowing Toy

Long-lasting

Jo Sweeney,
Hospital Play Specialist

Jo visited a Science Workshop in the USA where she watched children raising mounds of bubbles by this simple method. The top of a yoghurt pot was covered with a circle of terry towelling — held in place by a rubber band. A small hole was made in the side of the pot and a drinking straw inserted. After dipping the terry towelling top in bubble mixture, a child could blow through the straw. The more powerful his puff the higher the mound of bubbles he could raise! Jo adapted this idea to make a robust toy.

Materials
- A plastic cup from a set of stacking cups with a diameter of at least 5 cm (2"). The smaller the cup, the easier it is to build up enough pressure inside to raise the bubbles, so avoid the largest cups in the set.
- Terry towelling — an old face flannel will do.
- Shirring elastic — the thin, round kind used for gathering.
- Pony tail hairband — a small elasticated ring of soft fabric.
- A drinking straw.
- A drill bit slightly larger than the drinking straw.
- Bubble mixture, *see below*.

Method
Cut a circle of terry towelling to cover the top of the stacking cup and reach about half way down the side. Keep it in place with the pony tail band, and trim off any excess terry towelling. Thread a needle with shirring elastic and sew the pony tail hairband to the terry towelling with about two rows of running stitch. With the drill bit make a hole in the side of the stacking cup, just below the ponytail band. Dip the terry towelling top in bubble mixture. Insert a drinking straw in the hole and *blow*!

Note
If the bubble-blowing toy is to be used on another occasion by a different child, it is a simple matter to slide off and wash the terry towelling cap.

Recipe for Bubble Mixture

20 fl oz water
1 fl oz concentrated washing-up liquid
2 tablespoons glycerine (from the chemist)
Put all this in a plastic squash bottle and use as required.

TOYS TO ENCOURAGE LOOKING

When you first make the acquaintance of a new baby, what do you do? I guess you call his name, smile, nod your head, and generally make your face as noticeable as you can! It was Dr Elizabeth Newson, speaking at a toy library meeting several years ago, who made us realise that Mum (or Dad!) is the baby's first and best toy. The face of a caring adult has all the essentials—colour, movement, sound and *surprise*. The teeth appear, then hide; the tongue too; the eyes open and shut, and the mouth changes shape and makes odd noises like 'Boo!' Anything can happen! Pop-up toys also have all the essentials, plus a certain therapeutic value. Held by an adult, they can help a baby direct his gaze this way and that, up or down, left or right. When the child is able to hold the toy for himself, he will need to use both hands to make it work. While playing he should learn all about 'in' and 'out', and how to surprise people!

The following pop-up toys range from the ephemeral to the long-lasting. Try the best one for your child.

Pop-up Dolly

Instant

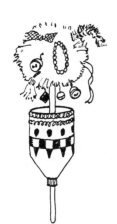

This is not a toy for a baby or toddler to *handle*. It is not robust and, if mouthed, could have disastrous consequences. However, it has great 'baby appeal' and is safe if *only* handled by an adult. Its virtue is that it really works, and can be made in a jiffy if you have the following materials handy.

Materials
- A washing-up liquid bottle.
- A dish mop.
- A promising collection of small items like bells, colourful buttons, large beads, lengths of ribbon, tinsel, etc. (This of course is the part that is dangerous for young children to handle.)
- A strip of Fablon, or Humbrol enamel (optional).

Method
Cut the plastic bottle in half. Remove the stopper and hold the top half of the bottle so that the neck points

downwards. Thread the handle of the mop through the neck. Tie the small items suggested above to the mop head. Perhaps wrap the bottle in Fablon, or paint it. This is an 'optional extra', but makes the dolly look more like a real toy than the collection of junk it really is!

To attract your baby's attention, all you now need to do is to make the mop pop out of the bottle and disappear inside again. By your own reactions, make this seem wildly exciting, and build up the suspense until the climax!

Pop-up Dolly
Safe Version
(For children to use on their own)

Quick

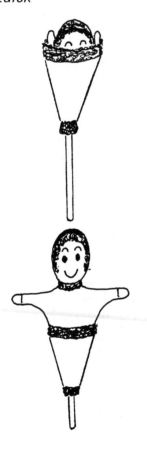

This toy is colourful and strong, and will withstand all but the most determined teethers.

Materials
- A wooden spoon. It *must* have a long handle if the dolly is to pop up properly.
- A cardboard or plastic cone from a spool of wool used on a knitting machine.
- Humbrol enamel in suitable colours for the face.
- A small piece of *thin* material for the dress.
- Thicker material to cover the cone.
- Scraps of trimming for decoration.
- PVA adhesive, needle and thread.

Method
Start by painting the face on the bowl of the spoon. Place the eyes in the middle and a smiley mouth below. Paint the back and inside edge of the bowl to represent hair. While the paint is drying, cut out the dress from the thin material. Fold it in half and cut out a shape like a flat letter T. Make sure that when the sides are sewn up, the bottom will be wide enough to fit comfortably round the top of the cone. Stitch up the side seams and turn the dress right side out. Cut out two small felt hands (as in the illustration), turn in the raw edges at the ends of the sleeves and sew in the hands. Now make a neck opening just large enough for the handle of the spoon to go through. Stick the dress to the spoon, just below the bowl. Use PVA adhesive generously and bind round the neck with cotton for extra strength and to prevent the dress

40

from pulling away from the neck before the adhesive has set. Thread the handle of the spoon down through the hole in the cone. Hold the dress round the outside of the lip of the cone. Check that the dolly completely disappears inside, and will pop up and down properly. You may have to shorten the skirt if it is too bulky, but beware of cutting away too much — a mini skirt will not allow the dolly to hide inside the cone. Stick the skirt securely to the lip of the cone and bind it with cotton as for the neck. Cover the cone with thick material. (Stick and/or sew.) Felt is ideal as it will not fray. For extra strength, it is worthwhile sewing the hem of the dress to the cover and neatening the join with velvet ribbon, or lampshade trimming etc. Embellish the neck with a ruff of gathered lace or ribbon.

Small Pop-up Dolly

Quick

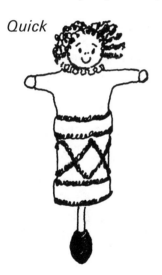

This version is basically the same as the safe pop-up dolly, but all the materials are scaled down. This makes it particularly suitable for 'frail' children, and for those with small hands. It is not for babies.

Materials
- A plastic film carton.
- Two wooden beads — one for the handle, the other for the head. The head can also be made from polyester fibre covered with material from a pair of tights.
- A short length of thin dowel, say 18 cm (7"), to fit the hole in the beads.
- Thin material for the dress.
- Thicker material to cover the carton.
- Bits and pieces for decoration — wool for hair, pink or brown felt for hands, lace for collar, etc.
- Felt pens or sewing cotton for the features.
- PVA adhesive, needle and thread.

Method
Prepare the carton by drilling a small hole in the centre of the bottom. Check that the dowel fits in it fairly loosely. Stick a natural wood bead to one end of the dowel, *or* make a soft head. Wrap a small amount of polyester fibre round the head of the dowel. Cover it

41

with a circle of double thickness tights material. Pull this tightly over the polyester fibre, squashing it into a nice round shape. Gather the material tightly round the dowel to make the neck. Try to smooth out the creases on the face side of the head. They do not matter at the back where they will be covered by hair or a hat. This is a fiddly job. I like to get the neck right by giving it a short binding of cotton, just to attach the head to the dowel, then I finish off the job with a liberal application of adhesive and more binding. This is the 'belt and braces' approach and should make sure the head will never pull off. Check that the head will fit *easily* in the carton. There must still be room for the dress. While the adhesive dries, cut out the dress as for the safe pop-up dolly, sew it up, insert the hands, make a small neck hole and try it for size. Tie it temporarily round the neck, poke the dowel down through the hole in the carton, hold the hem to the lip and have a trial run. If all goes well, stick and bind the dress to the neck. Stick and bind the hem of the dress to the lip of the carton. Cover the carton, and stick a bead on the end of the dowel. Finally add the embellishments — the features, hair, hat?, collar, and trimming for the carton.

Miniature Pop-up Dolly

Very Quick

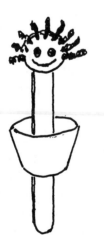

This little toy is small enough to slip into a pocket or handbag. It is so simple to make that even older children can have a go. At the toy library we have a little stock in reserve for emergencies. They are useful as a tiny gift for a birthday child, or to welcome a new member. One has even been known to surprise a child in the middle of a temper tantrum and stop a rumpus!

Materials
- A lolly stick.
- A section from an egg box.
- A button.
- Glue — U-Hu or other clear glue (for plastics) is best.

Method
Stick the button to one end of the lolly stick. Mark a face on it with felt pen and add some wool hair.

Make a slit in the bottom of the egg box section and poke the lolly stick through it. Now all you have to do is to slide the lolly stick up and down to make the button face appear, then hide in the egg box section. To hide its humble origins, this can of course be decorated.

Tunnel Pop-up Toy

Quick

Marianne Willemsen-van Witsen

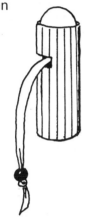

This toy can be fun for lots of children — the very active as well as the not so mobile. A ping-pong ball is hidden inside a tube. A sharp pull on the ribbon projects it out of the top — to be chased all over the room by the energetic. Pull the ribbon more gently to make the ball pop out less dramatically and a skilful child, perhaps in a wheelchair, might be able to catch it before it reaches the floor.

Materials
- A ping-pong ball.
- A cardboard tube. Check that the tube is *slightly* wider than the ping-pong ball, for this has to move freely up and down inside it.
- Soft ribbon, about $2\frac{1}{2}$ cm (1″) wide and roughly four times the length of the tube.
- A bead for the end of the ribbon. This is optional, but makes it easier to grasp.
- PVA adhesive.
- Scissors (or a craft knife for adult use.)
- Decoration for the tube — paint, paper, Fablon or cloth.

Method
Cut a horizontal slit, like a letter box, in the cardboard tube, fairly near the top. Make it wide enough for the ribbon to slide through easily. Thread the ribbon through the slot to the inside of the tube. Pull it up and away from you so that it comes out of the tube and over the edge. Stick it down the entire length of the 'back' of the tube. This will attach it firmly so that it will withstand plenty of pulling. Thread the free end of the ribbon through the bead and tie a knot.

Once the glue is dry, the toy is almost finished and ready for its trials. Try it out by pushing the ping-pong ball down inside the tube. It will sit in the sling of the ribbon. Pull the ribbon smartly, and the ball should shoot out of the top of the tube. If you have a problem, it could be because the tube has been slightly squashed, and the ball gets stuck. Reinforce the tube with strips of paper and glue, or find another one and start again! Perhaps the slot needs enlarging slightly, or even moving a little nearer the top of the tube.

When you are satisfied the toy is working well, decorate the tube.

Pop-up Matchbox

Quick

Marianne Willemsen-van Witsen

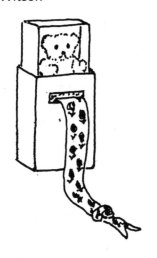

If you have already made the Tunnel Pop-up Toy you will have no difficulty with this one. It works on the same principle, but the action is slower and less dramatic. Pull the ribbon, and the tray of the matchbox will rise most of the way out of its cover to reveal its hidden treasure.

Materials
- A matchbox.
- A short length of ribbon, about 2 cm ($\frac{3}{4}''$) wide.
- A bead (optional).
- A decorative cover for the matchbox.
- Something to stick inside for the surprise — a tiny doll, a toy from a cracker, or perhaps a familiar face cut from a photograph. If you have time and the inclination, you might create a little scene inside the tray, such as a window looking out onto a country scene, with dainty lace curtains and pot plants on the window sill.

Method
Remove the tray from the matchbox cover. Cut a slot about 2 cm from the top of the cover (wide enough to take the ribbon). If you make it nearer the top, the tray will come right out when the ribbon is pulled. If you make it further down, not enough of the tray will rise up. Even making a simple little toy like this can have its technical hazards.

Thread the ribbon through the slot to the inside of the cover, and pull it up and over the back. Stick it along the entire length of the back. Insert the tray gently so that it sits in the ribbon sling, then press it down. (The ribbon will shorten as the tray disappears inside the cover.) Tie a bead to the free end of the ribbon. Pull it gently to make sure the top is working properly and the tray rises up as you expect.

Take the tray out and decorate the part that will show. Then decorate the cover — the quickest way is to wrap it in coloured Sellotape, and this will also cover the abrasive strips at the side.

Jumping Jacks

Long-lasting

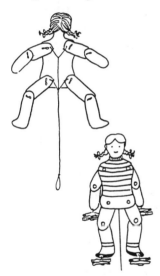

Jumping Jacks are traditional toys, usually made in wood. This version is in cardboard. It combines movement with sound, and is jointed with paper fasteners — the kind with 'legs' that open out.

It is sensible to make a paper pattern first. This can help you to decide on the size and the shape of the pieces, and you can make sure your design will work well before you spend time on the cardboard version.

Before you begin, look at the illustration and work out the mechanics of making your Jack (or Jill) jump. Then draw the body with the head attached by a fairly thick neck (for strength). Cut out two sausage-shaped arms and decide on the best positions for them. They must swivel on the paper fasteners so as to be horizontal with the body when the connecting string is pulled fully down, and be almost hidden by the body when relaxed. Cut out the legs, also sausage-shaped, but larger than the arms and with suggested feet on the end. When you are happy with your design, transfer the shapes to fairly thick cardboard and cut them out with a craft knife or Snips (really strong kitchen scissors similar to secateurs). Paint all the pieces. Fix on the limbs with paper fasteners, and string them as shown in the illustration. For an added attraction, tie a string of foil milk-bottle tops (with a button on the bottom of the string to stop them slipping off), to the hands and feet. Alternatively, tie on bells.

Hang your Jumping Jack against a plain wall if possible, and just out of a child's reach, so that the string must be pulled to make him dance.

Plywood Owl Jumping Jack

Long-lasting

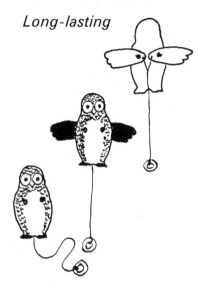

This toy works on the same principle as the one above, but only his wings move. For anyone with a fretsaw it is easy to make, and the finished owl is very robust.

Make a paper pattern first. Draw the owl's head and body, making him about 30 cm (12") long. Give him large eyes and make him chubby so that his wings will fold neatly behind his body when at rest. Draw his wings and try them out by fixing them in place with paper clips. Make sure they will flap nicely. Transfer the body and wing shapes to the plywood and cut them out. Sandpaper all the parts and paint in the eyes, beak and feathers. Drill two holes in each wing, one to fix it to the body and the other near the edge for the pull string. I joined my wings to the body with piping cord, knotting it in front of the body and behind the wings. Small nuts and bolts or rivets could be used. String up as shown in the illustration.

Note
After several weeks of heavy use, the piping cord on my owl stretched, and the wings started to rotate (!) causing a tangle at the back. Should this happen to you, the remedy is easy. Just glue a small strip of wood across the owl's shoulders to act as a stop.

Straw Dancing Dolly

Quick

Pam Rigley,
Toymaker

This energetic little doll makes a delightful novelty toy. It is soon made from plastic drinking straws and beads — all held together with button thread. With the help of gravity, it can be made to dance like a tiny puppet and its bead feet will tap out a tattoo on the table top. It is attractive to many children but, because of its tiny size and light weight, it is particularly suitable for 'frail' ones.

Materials
- Plastic drinking straws.
- A bead for the head (or a cotton ball as shown in the illustration).
- Four smaller beads for the hands and feet.
- Button thread.

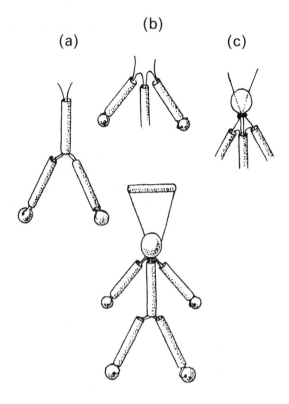

Method

First cut the drinking straws the right size to represent the body, arms and legs. Cut a long piece of button thread, and begin at the neck. Pass the thread down the body, then down one leg, through a bead on the foot, and back up the leg. Now carry on with the other leg. Pass the thread down it, through the bead for the foot, back up the leg and through the body. Hopefully you now have two threads emerging from the neck end (a). Use one for threading up each arm — down the straw, through the bead and back up the straw (b). Knot the arm threads together, then pass them through the head bead or, if you are using a cotton ball, thread them through with a needle (c). Make a dangle handle from a small piece of drinking straw. Finish off by passing one thread through the dangle handle and knot it to the end of the other. Hold the doll by the handle and dangle her about. The weight of the beads on her hands and feet will help her to dance with abandon.

A Peep-bo Toy

Quick

Catherine O'Neil,
Speech Therapist and
Toy Maker

This toy is a cross between a pop-up toy and a jumping jack. The surprise element works on the lever principle. When the string is pulled, a picture pops out from behind a bunch of colourful balloons.

The dotted lines on the illustration show how it works.

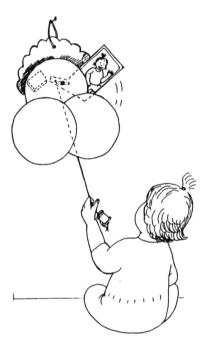

Materials
- Cardboard for the backing circle, balloons and picture holder.
- Felt pens or paint.
- A paper fastener with legs.
- A matchbox to act as a spacer, or several strips of cardboard stuck together to make an equivalent shape.
- A pull string with a cotton reel on the end.
- Photographs or pictures for the surprise.

Method
Make the backing circle in cardboard. Draw round a dinner plate and scallop one edge, as in the illustration, to add to the artistic effect. Paint in white. Cut out three more cardboard circles, about the size of tea plates, and colour them in primary colours. Cut out the picture holder. Make it about 10×16 cm ($4 \times 6\frac{1}{2}''$) — the right size for a photograph or picture post card — and allow for the 'tail' to make it work (*see* illustration.) Make two small holes in the tail for the pull string and the paper fastener. Tie on the pull string. Fix the picture holder to the backing card with the paper fastener and test that it will pop up and down easily. If it sticks, *slightly* enlarge the hole. Stick the matchbox — or laminated cardboard spacer — to the backing card. Stick one circle to the matchbox. Stick the other two circles on top, making sure they will cover the picture holder when 'at rest', and that the picture will pop out properly when the string is pulled. Fix the picture to the holder. Consider using Blu-tac if you want to change it often. Hang up the Peep-bo toy so that only the pull string is within reach of the child. If his reaction is true to form, his new toy will both attract and capture his attention.

A Peep-bo Puppet

Almost Instant

Mme Schneider

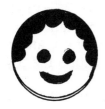

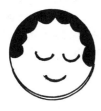

Mme Schneider lives in Switzerland and is a teacher of visually impaired children. She finds this 'high contrast' little puppet ideal for a quick game of Peep-bo. She claims it is made in a jiffy, and she is right!

Cut two circles of white material, about the size of a saucer. Stitch or stick them together for just over half way round, leaving an opening at the bottom for your hand. Slip some stiff paper (or card) between the circles to prevent the ink from spreading through, and draw a face on both sides with a black marker pen. Perhaps one face could be happy and the other sad, or one awake and the other asleep. Draw some black hair round the top of the face. Remove the paper, put your hand inside, and show the puppet to your child. Now you are ready for a game of Peep-bo. Make the little face pop out from behind the curtain, or suddenly appear over the top of the arm chair.

Visi-bottles

What happens to your empty bubblebath bottle before it lands up in the dustbin? In our house, I used to half fill it with water and give it to our energetic little two-year-old. He would use it like a cocktail shaker to build up an impressive head of bubbles inside the bottle, then watch intently as they gradually popped, restoring the water to its previous state and ready for its next frantic shake up. Over the years the idea of using a plastic bottle with different contents developed into the creation of the 'Visi bottle'. Perhaps it is the feeling of movement and weight as the water sloshes about inside, or maybe it is the gentle and controllable rearrangement of the contents that gives it child appeal. Even children for whom other toys seem to hold little interest sometimes respond to this type of toy. For very little effort and no expense it can certainly make a useful addition to a collection of toys to watch.

A Visi-bottle to Shake

Do you remember the 'snowstorm' toys that were popular a few years ago? They can still be found occasionally in gift shops. A water-filled dome of clear plastic covers a tiny winter scene. Turn the toy upside down, then right way up and 'snowflakes' gently flutter through the water to settle over the scene.

A cheap and cheerful variation of this toy can be made in a jiffy. Fill a clear plastic bottle with water, sprinkle in a small amount of desiccated coconut or some oats and tightly screw on the cap. Give the bottle a quick shake to stir up the contents, then watch the particles slowly sink to the bottom. The water tends to become cloudy eventually, but by then the toy will probably have lost its appeal.

An improved version can be made by filling a small clear plastic bottle with glycerine (from the chemist) and using silver glitter for the snow. These materials are more expensive, but may be worth it. The bottle can make an attractive ephemeral toy, perhaps for a 'frail' child who needs a low-effort plaything.

A Swishing Jar

Very quick

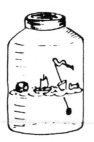

I first made this toy for a lively three-year-old who had both a hearing and a sight impairment. He was a 'wanderer'. It was difficult to persuade him to sit at the table and play with a toy even for a brief spell. Most playthings soon ended up on the floor. Not so the Swishing Jar! It was *large* and *heavy* and quite different from all the normal brightly coloured plastic toys he was usually offered. He would sit with his nose nearly touching the jar as he rocked it and watched the floating objects bob about on the surface of the water. When he was tired of looking at the ping-pong ball, corks and cotton reel, they could be exchanged for a tiny boat, some chips of polystyrene packaging or any other flotsam that happened to be to hand.

You can see from the illustration that the Swishing Jar is a converted sweet jar — the kind that, a few years ago, might be thrown away by the owner of the sweet shop on the corner. They are still occasionally available from this source, but these days you may have to buy a plastic storage jar. If you make this toy for a child whose hands are large enough to unscrew the top, fix it in place with U-Hu or other plastic glue. This will avoid unwanted spillage but, of course, the contents of the bottle cannot be changed.

Egg-timer Bottles

Quick

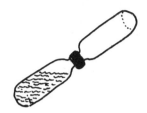

I remember first seeing this toy at an adventure playground and watching two children being fascinated by it for a considerable time. It turns up in schools, playgroups and playschemes, which proves its popularity with the children. If you fancy making one, find two plastic bottles with the same sized necks. Nearly fill one with water and add a few drops of food colouring. Join the necks together with a plastic glue, U-Hu or similar. When the glue has set, bind the join securely with plastic sticky tape (parcel tape or electrician's tape).

As an alternative filling, try a fine, dry substance as in a real egg-timer. Sand, rice, even fine fish grit will not clog, and could be safe in the event of the bottles coming apart.

A Visi-tube

Quick

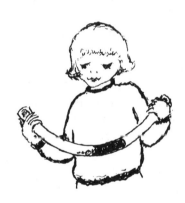

I invented this plaything when working as a toymaker in one school for children with severe learning difficulties. One of the teachers had requested a toy to help a particular boy. This lad had difficulty in holding an object with both hands, and usually opted out by only using his 'good' one. The more often he was able to solve his problems this way, the less likely he was to be able to make use of his 'lazy' hand. My first Visi-tube was an attempt to help him use both together. It would only work if held that way. It consisted of about 1 m (40") of tough, clear, thick plastic tubing as used in home wine-making. One end of the tube was blocked off by ramming a cork well inside the rim, so that the only way of removing it would be with a corkscrew. Brightly coloured beads, tiny buttons etc. small enough to slide easily along the tube without getting jammed were fed into the open end of the tube. Then this was corked up. The idea was to hold the tube at both ends, then tilt it by alternately raising and lowering each hand, so making the contents in the tube race from one end to the other and back again. The boy managed to make the beads move a little at the first try and was motivated gradually to improve his skill.

In the class was another boy who was reluctant to hold anything at all. After watching his friend play, he consented to hold one end of the Visi-tube while his teacher held the other. He cottoned on to the idea of rolling the beads from his end to hers by raising his arm, but it took some time for him to realise he must lower it to make them roll back again.

The rest of the class soon wanted to play too, and queued up to take turns. We encouraged more concentrated looking by masking off a section of the tube with opaque sticky tape. The boys learnt how to control the tube so that the contents could be hidden behind the tape.

I have since made slightly shorter Visi-tubes for a few of our toy library members. Emma, a four-year-old who also had difficulty in using both hands, had extra fun with hers. She was an articulate little girl and together we made up little stories to help her to control the tube. Perhaps the beads represented a train that must stop in the station — the masked-off section of the tube. The passengers were cross if some of the carriages were left outside and they couldn't alight! Maybe the beads were 'children' out for a leisurely walk when all of a sudden the rain fell down and they must scuttle for shelter behind the tape. Sometimes the beads were tipped beyond the shelter and the children got wet. (Giggles from Emma!)

This toy is virtually indestructible and therefore can be suitable for 'tough guys'. It is not for use by an unsupervised rumbustious group. It might be swung about by one end and used as a weapon!

Scrapbooks

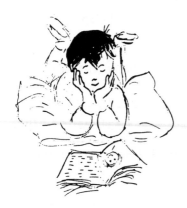

These can be very personal possessions when made for a particular child, and can often hold his attention when all other books fail. If you have not yet made a scrapbook, you may find the following hints helpful:

1. *Make the subject of your book topical*
   Children are primarily interested in everything that directly concerns themselves, and a book entitled 'Me' can be a winner! The pages could include photos of the child and his family, and pictures of his favourite toys, his chosen make of car, pets, favourite food, picture postcards, tickets saved from

an outing — even the wrapping from a bar of chocolate can have special significance.

2. *Keep the book short*
A child who is just old enough to enjoy a scrapbook is likely to have a limited span of attention, and may still be at the tearing stage. It is better to spend the time making four thin books than one magnificent fat one. This way the books can have more variety and, should the temptation to tear become overwhelming, it is not as disastrous as the destruction of a large book would be.

3. *Use the strongest and most colourful materials*
Plain wallpaper (not the bumpy kind or vinyl coated, or the scraps will not stick properly) can be pasted onto card from cartons — cereal packets, washing powder boxes, etc. — to make the pages of a board book. These pages can be tied together loosely in three places so that they will turn over easily. Pages can also be cut from thick brown paper and stitched together. Coloured sticky tape can be used to reinforce the edges, and this will also cheer up the brown paper.

4. *Make sure the edges of the scraps are well stuck down* or the temptation to 'pick' will be irresistible!

Note
If you have taken the trouble to make a special scrapbook, it will be disappointing if it is soon torn. Look at it during a quiet moment when you can talk about the pictures and savour them together. The book could be a firm favourite and subject to heavy wear. It may be worthwhile protecting the pages with clear sticky-backed plastic (from a large stationer's shop). A special scrapbook that has taken time and effort to make may well become a family treasure and be worth preserving.

A Scrap Sheet

Instant

This is just a large sheet of paper fixed to the wall or the back of a door. It must be at the right height for the child to see properly, and to be able to point to the pictures. Every day a new one can be added until there is no more room.

A Zigzag Scrapbook

Quick

This makes a change from the conventional scrapbook, and can be made to stand up so that the child can see all the pictures in a long line. Stiff paper or thin card is folded zigzag fashion so that it can close up and open out like a concertina. Pictures can be stuck to both sides. A good subject for this kind of book might be 'In the Street'. Pictures of cars, lorries, a fire engine, an ambulance, a bus, a removal van, bicycles, people, etc. could be pasted on each section of the book. When opened out, it will show a long picture like a frieze.

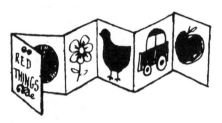

Rag Books

Long-lasting

Rag books for young children have undoubted advantages over paper ones. The pages are thick and easy to turn. They are virtually untearable and can be dribbled on — even chewed — and then restored to their first glory by a quick swirl in the washing machine.

If your child is at the rag book stage, but is not attracted by commercial ones, this may be because the pictures are too small for him to see properly, or are cluttered up with words, or are just not about things that interest him. Why not try making him a special one?

Materials
- Plain material for the pages. Unbleached calico is best. It is strong and cheap.
- Nursery curtaining for the pictures. This is usually printed in bold colours and has clear pictures, which make excellent illustrations for a rag book. Search around fabric shops, market stalls, jumble sales and car boot sales (for second-hand curtains), and you will find a choice of animals, nursery

rhymes, spacemen, cartoon characters and many more.
- A sewing machine.

Method

Decide on the size of your proposed book, then cut the plain material into pieces twice as wide as each page. Each piece will be doubled over, so that the fold makes the turning edge of the page. Cut out the pictures you have chosen, leaving a narrow border round the edge for the stitching. Using a very narrow machine stitch, attach two pictures to every piece of material, one each side of the fold. Change to a narrow zigzag stitch and sew round them all again. To make up the pages, put the pictures face to face, and straight stitch along the top and bottom of each page. You have now made a bag. The open side will become the spine of the book. Turn the bag inside out, so that the pictures now show. Press each page, and sew them all together at the open ends. They will probably be too thick to go under the machine. I join two or three by machine, then oversew them all with button thread. A strip of material sewn over the spine will cover the raw edges and make the book look neater.

If you enjoy sewing, it can be rewarding to make the pictures as a collage of your own design, perhaps incorporating a variety of textures. This kind of book makes a good present. It is washable, and well worth making for a toy library or hospital play scheme, where it can be enjoyed by a succession of children.

Picture Window Rag Books

Long-lasting

Every factory-made rag book is designed for babies. It is impossible to find one suitable for an older child with learning difficulties or hand function problems. The Picture Window Rag Book is unique, because it includes all the advantages of easily turned pages, indestructibility and washability (at a low temperature) *and* it can be made interesting for a child of any age —just like the family photograph album.

Each page is empty, except for a clear plastic window stitched down on three sides. The fourth side is left free so the photograph, picture postcard or any other pictures of the same size can be inserted between the page and the plastic window. By this simple method the pictures can be changed as often as necessary. One week, perhaps, the book will feature photos of the family and pets. These might be replaced by pictures of vehicles and street scenes, to be followed by photographic memories of a school trip.

I have made several of these books for individual children, each with special needs. One was for a girl of eleven. She could not walk without support and was unable to speak. She was also partially sighted. My aim was to try to widen the scope of her playtime by offering her an alternative to shaking various noisemakers or banging two toys together. Her book contained six pages. The pictures needed to be large, so the windows were made 20 × 20 cm (8 × 8″). They were stitched to the right hand pages only. I felt this would make it easier for her to learn to turn the pages over. I drew large, clear pictures of her toys and clothes, her family car and her wheelchair. I also made a few extra pages from black paper, and decorated them with diffraction stickers bought off the roll at a local toy shop. On a bright day, these showed up brilliantly in the sunlight and gave her particular pleasure.

Another book was made when my little friend Rupert was two years old. He had a skin problem, and his toys needed to be soft to avoid friction and, of course, they were washed frequently to keep them hygienic. His book contained ten pages, and there was a window on both sides. Each window measured 17 × 12 cm ($6\frac{3}{4}$ × $4\frac{3}{4}$″), the right size to hold a photograph or a picture postcard. His illustrations were of people he knew, and of parts of his village, plus some specially made ones to help him to recognise colours and to count. (A bunch of balloons and a collection of pairs of shoes, to name but two examples.)

If you decide to make a Picture Window Rag Book, first ask yourself how many pages it should have, and then what size the pictures should be. Then consult the 'shopping list' below.

Materials
- Fabric for the pages. Unbleached calico is best.

- Plastic material for the windows. I used PVC from the soft furnishing department of a large store. The plastic must be pliable, for it must accept machine stitching, and be able to bend when the pages are turned inside out.
- Black tape, or black bias binding for the frames.
- Plenty of pictures. Collect several sets the same size, so that they can be easily interchanged.

Method

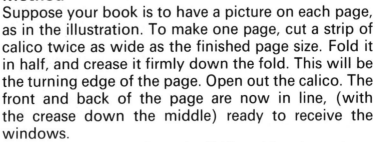

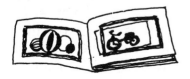

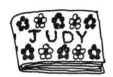

Suppose your book is to have a picture on each page, as in the illustration. To make one page, cut a strip of calico twice as wide as the finished page size. Fold it in half, and crease it firmly down the fold. This will be the turning edge of the page. Open out the calico. The front and back of the page are now in line, (with the crease down the middle) ready to receive the windows.

Cut two windows from the PVC, making them about 1cm wider all round than the pictures they will cover. Make the frames from the tape. Cut it into lengths corresponding to the sides of the windows, allowing a little extra for tucking under at the corners. Position the tape on three sides of the window, so that about half overlaps the edge of the PVC. Sew it to the PVC with a single row of stitching. On the fourth side (the one that is to be left unattached to the page) bind the tape round the PVC and attach it with two rows of stitching. Now sew the frames to the page. Arrange for the open ends to face the spine. This will make it more difficult for the children to remove the pictures or for them to fall out accidentally. Pin the other three sides to the page and stitch them in position. Fold the front and back of the page together with the frames face to face. Stitch along the top and bottom edges, making a bag with the spine side open. Turn the bag right side out. Lightly press the *edges*. Avoid the PVC, of course, or you will melt it — and have a very messy iron to clean! Make as many similar pages as you want.

Make a front and back cover very slightly larger than the pages. There is a chance to embroider or applique a design here, or you can go for the easy option and use a pretty fabric. Join the pages and covers together in pairs, with the machine, then oversew the lot with button thread. Cover the spine with ribbon, a strip of fabric or braid, to hide the raw edges and the oversewing.

A Counting Book for Yasmeen

Long-lasting

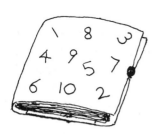

Yasmeen is a very intelligent three-year-old. Sadly she has an illness that confines her to a chair and restricts the use of her arms. She needs tabletop toys that are small, light and intellectually challenging. One of her favourite toys is her counting book that also doubles up as a picture book. It is made on the same principle as the rag book and the picture window book described above, but bearing in mind Yasmeen's special needs, the pages are considerably smaller. (Actual size 10 × 15 cm, 4 × 6".) A flap is attached to the bottom edges of the front and back covers. Each flap holds five numbers, embroidered on small felt circles and attached by Velcro spots. Every page of the book is decorated with items to count. The required number is lifted from the flap and transferred to the Velcro spot on the page. The flaps tuck in when the book is not in use, and the pages are kept closed with a small button and loop.

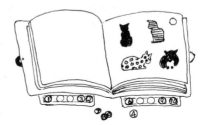

It took many evenings to make the book, but I think the time was well spent. The result was an unusual and special present for a 'frail' child. I have since made another for Rupert, and I am sure that will not be the last — this is one of those toys where the creator has as much fun as the recipient!

Here are the ideas I used for the pages — just to start you thinking.

- *One felt house* — with embroidered window boxes and roses round the door. A face looks out of the window, and a cat sits sunning itself on the doorstep. (All embroidered.)

- *Two fish with black sequin eyes* — cut from glamorous gold and silver material and appliqued on to the page.
- *Three little faces* — made in stockinette and slightly padded from the back to give them shape. (Trepunto quilting.) The hair is made from wool: French knots for curls, straight for plaits. I stitched boys' haircuts for Rupert's book. (Yasmeen holds little conversations with her faces.)
- *Four cats* — cut from felt, and suitably embellished.
- *Five sequin flowers* in a felt bowl.
- *Six buttons* on a felt coat.
- *A bunch of seven felt balloons*.
- *Eight ribbon roses* on a rosebush.
- *Nine sequin stars* on a dark blue felt sky.
- *Ten small wooden beads* on a necklace. (For Rupert, a man about to climb a ladder with ten rungs.)

Cup and Ball

Quick

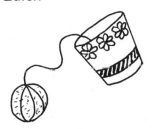

This traditional toy has given pleasure to children down the ages. It is pictured on an ancient Greek vase, and we know the little daughter of Marie Antoinette had one exquisitely carved in ivory, called a bilboquet. It was a favourite in Victorian nurseries and still turns up in a wooden form in gift shops and craft markets.

The toy consists of a ball attached to a cup by a fairly long string. The aim is to swing the ball and catch it in the cup. This is not as easy as it would appear! As a 'watching toy' it has its uses — take your eye off the ball and it is sure to miss the cup! It does not take long to make a simple version suitable for young children and those with limited dexterity.

Make the ball soft, so that if it flies into the child's face, it will do no damage. Either make a woolly ball, or fashion it out of crunched–up newspaper.

Materials
- For the ball, either cardboard and brightly coloured wool, or newspaper and kitchen foil.
- Button thread or thin string.

- A yoghurt pot for the cup. (If a handle is necessary, use the top half of a washing-up liquid bottle. Make a short handle from dowel to fit the neck, and glue it in place.)
- Optional extra. Fablon or felt and trimming (stuck or sewn) to decorate the cup.

Method

To make a woolly ball, cut two identical circles from card, e.g. from a Cornflakes packet, diameter about 4 cm ($1\frac{3}{4}''$). Cut a hole in the centre of each, about $1\frac{1}{2}$ cm ($\frac{3}{4}''$). Put the circles together and wind the wool over the edge and up through the middle, gradually working your way round the ring. At this stage the ball resembles a ring doughnut. As the hole fills up you will need a needle to finish the winding. If you hold the ring up to your eye you should not be able to see through it. Take a sharp pair of pointed scissors and, at one place on the circumference of the circle, snip the wool until you come to the cardboard. Then poke the scissors between the pieces of card and continue cutting all round. You now have lots of strands of wool sticking out each side of the cardboard circles. Part the cardboard circles a little way. Using button thread *tightly* wind round the wool between the cardboard circles, finishing off with a sturdy knot. Tie the attaching string firmly in the same place, i.e. between the cardboard circles, then snip them and pull them away. Fluff up the wool to make the ball a good shape and trim off any odd ends. Make sure the ball will fit in the yoghurt pot. If not, trim it again.

To make a newspaper ball, tightly crunch half a sheet, or a whole one from a tabloid. Check that it will fit in the yoghurt pot. Wrap kitchen foil round it to give it some sparkle and glamour. Keep it a good shape by binding round it once with button thread or thin string, and tie the ends together. Then continue binding tightly round the ball, as if making lines of longitude on the globe! Tie the ends together again and attach the joining string.

Decorate the yoghurt pot if you wish. Make a small hole near the rim — or in the centre of the bottom — it does not seem to matter which you choose. Tie the ball to the yoghurt pot. Use a short string for beginners, or a longer string for the more confident ones.

Little Tumbling Men

Quick

This is a traditional toy sometimes found at craft markets or gift shops. It is a superb tracking toy, and the sight of the little man somersaulting down a slope never fails to excite both children and the adults caring for them.

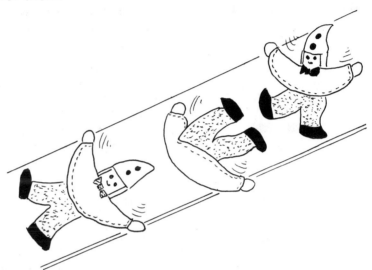

Many people have asked me for the pattern, so here goes ....

Materials
- A plastic film carton.
- A tool for removing the bottom and rim — small hack saw, or craft knife.
- A marble — as large as possible, but it must fit *easily* inside the carton.
- Scraps of felt — bright colours, with perhaps a little black for contrast.
- PVA adhesive.
- Needle and cotton.

Method
Cut off the rim and bottom of the film carton, converting it into a tube. For the face, cut off a small strip of felt (pink or brown), long enough to cover about half the tube, and wide enough to wrap

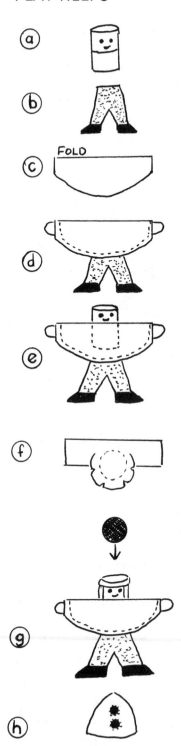

(a)

(b)

(c) FOLD

(d)

(e)

(f)

(g)

(h)

completely round it. Make the features—embroider them or use tiny felt circles stitched on. Stick the face to the tube, as in illustration (a). While the adhesive is drying, cut out the legs and feet in single felt (b). Shoes are an optional extra. Cut out the jacket from folded felt (c). Cut out two small hands and pin them to the ends of the arms. Pin the legs in position. Stab stitch all these pieces to the jacket (d). Cut a slit in the top centre of the jacket, just large enough to take the tube. Smear the bottom half of the tube fairly liberally with adhesive and insert it into the jacket. Press the two together and hold them in position to give the adhesive a chance to stick (e). Cut out the head piece as in the illustration (f). It must be able to cover the top of the tube and overlap the forehead, back and sides of the tube. *Put in the marble*! Now cover the top of the tube with the head piece (g). It sometimes needs a bit of jiggery pokery to make it fit. I find it best to spread adhesive on the man's forehead, then round the back and sides of his head, and temporally bind the head piece in place with cotton. This holds the felt surfaces together while the adhesive sets. Cut out the hat in single felt (h). Sew felt spots or sequins to it. (If you only stick them on they will not survive many tumbles.) Remove the cotton binding from the head. Stick the hat to the front of the head piece (i), and again bind it with cotton until the adhesive sets. Neaten the join between the face and jacket by stitching on a felt collar or a bow tie.

Of course, the little tumbling man needs a sloping surface for his acrobatics. A piece of board covered with felt and propped up on a few books works well; so does an ironing board, closed flat, covered with a blanket and inclined to make the required slope.

(i)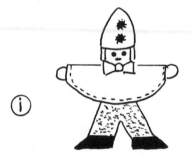

LEARNING TO IDENTIFY COLOURS

The development of language happens quite naturally with most children, and the names of colours are added, bit by bit, to their ever-widening vocabularies. All they seem to need are references to their *blue* mug, or *yellow* wellies and they 'catch on'. Other children are not so fortunate and may need many opportunities to practise identifying and naming colours.

For all children, colour matching games can be fun, and are usually the first step to more complicated ones. If your child needs practise in matching and naming colours, you may find among the following an activity or game that could be useful.

A cautionary tale! I remember vividly a frustrating afternoon, many years ago, spent with a boy at the hospital school where I then worked. I was using the Colour Matching Mat (p. 68) with him and he was having less than 50% success. He was putting the objects anywhere. I had not expected this as he was one of the more able pupils. Was he bored, or just playing up? A thought struck me and I asked one of the nurses if he was colour blind. 'Yes,' she replied. She must have had fun watching me struggle all afternoon. If you draw a blank with colour matching games, this might be the reason. Go for shape matching instead.

Colour Sorter

Instant

There are occasions when a busy adult can be desperate for an instant occupation for an equally busy child! Perhaps this simple idea is worth a try.

Find an empty egg box, apple tray or any item of throw-away packaging that contains divisions, and get out your button box. The challenge for the child is to sort the buttons by colour into the various compartments. Some buttons are bound to wander, so put everything on a tray.

Dress the Twins

Quick

Catherine O'Neil

Catherine uses two teddy bears for her colour matching activity. The idea is to dress the teddies alike. At the simplest level they can wear necklaces of identical beads. Ideally these are threaded by the child, and beads of only one colour are selected from the box. If beads are not handy, coloured plastic drinking straws

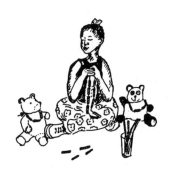

Fashion Coordinates

Quick

Chemene Hoare

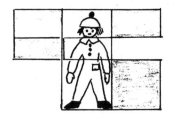

can be cut into short lengths and threaded onto pipe cleaners (for small teddies!) or shoelaces. The teddies can also be dressed in matching clothes. A square of felt with a hole in the middle will pass for a poncho, and a bobble hat and scarf can be knitted to match. For children with nimble fingers, more sophisticated clothes can be made. These might include Velcro or button fastenings. Obviously, several sets of clothes are required so that the child must make a choice.

With a little ingenuity you can make a figure of a child with interchangeable outfits. All you need is a sheet of card, or stiff paper, and three felt pens, say red, blue and yellow. This toy is popular with 'frail' children, and has its uses with others. It is a novel way of reinforcing colour recognition and naming.

Mark out the card into three equal columns. Fold in the side columns to cover the central one. Open out the card. Draw a child — head, body and legs — to fill the middle section. With horizontal cuts, divide each side piece into three flaps which will correspond to the head, the body and the legs of the central figure. (The head flap will be narrower than the others.) Fold in the top flap on the left hand side so that it covers the central head. On it draw a new head, making sure it lines up with the central body. Fold in the left hand middle flap. Draw another body to line up with the new head and the original legs. Finish off the new person by folding in the bottom flap and drawing the legs. Repeat the process with the three right hand flaps.

Now for the colourful part. The central figure might wear, say, a red hat, yellow jersey and blue skirt (or trousers!). The figure on the left could have a yellow hat, blue jersey and red bottom half, while the one on the right wears blue on top, red in the middle and yellow at the bottom. Puzzle — fold the card this way and that until the clothes of each person are entirely one colour.

Note
Another way of using this card is to draw three different characters across the columns. Bear in mind the

64

interests of the child you are aiming to entertain and draw the figures accordingly. Let your imagination wander too far and you may end up with a ballet dancer wearing a bowler hat and football boots!

Colour Dominoes

Quick

The summer holidays were approaching and one of the toy library families was heading for a caravan holiday. The weather forecast was not promising, so Mum made a hasty visit to the toy library to stock up on wet weather activities that could come in handy in a restricted space. On the 'Help Yourself' table were some kits for making a personal set of colour dominoes. I had used the idea when our children were young, and it came in useful again in this situation.

Each kit consisted of lots of card oblongs and several sheets of large, circular, white Blick Labels, which are sold in packs at many stationers. The idea was that children could colour the labels with a set of felt pens — only two of each colour — then peel them off the backing paper and stick them appropriately to the card oblongs to create a set of simple colour matching dominoes. The easiest way of making sure the colours match up correctly is to lay all the card oblongs out in a row, like the carriages in a train. Leave half of the first card blank, then for example stick a red circle to the other half. The other red circle goes on the first half of the next card, and a new colour is stuck to the other half .... and so on all down the line, ending with a blank.

Colour Peg Tin

Long-lasting

This toy seems to attract all young children. Toddlers love the clatter the pegs make when they are stirred around in the tin. They are good to chew too! Before long, they cotton on to the idea of placing them on the rim of the tin — unwittingly practising their hand-eye coordination! The older ones use the toy properly and match all the pegs to the appropriate sides of the

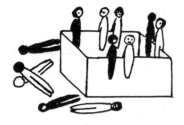

tin. As an added adult attraction, the toy makes its own container. At clearing-up time, all that needs to be done is to put the pegs inside and pop on the lid.

Materials
- A deep, square biscuit tin.
- About 48 wooden dolly pegs as in the illustration. These are still available at country ironmongers and, sometimes at street markets, kitchen shops, etc. Buy when you see them.
- Humbrol enamel in four colours.
- Small paint brush and white spirit for cleaning.
- Black fibre-tipped pen for the faces.
- Polyurethane varnish.
- Cardboard carton — useful for holding the pegs while they dry.

Method
Mark two diagonal lines across the inside of the bottom of the tin. You now have four triangles. Start by painting one of the triangles, say red: also the adjacent side, both inside and out. While waiting for the tin to dry, start on the peg men. Draw a face on every knob with the fibre pen: two dots for eyes and a smiley mouth. Take twelve pegs and give them red hats and bodies to match the side of the tin you have just finished. Fit the pegs over the side of the carton so that their legs can be painted without you having to hold them. Paint another side of the tin, outside, inside and bottom triangle as before, and paint the next twelve men to match... and so on. When the paint is dry, dip all the heads in polyurethane varnish to prevent the little faces from being rubbed off with handling, and brush the varnish over the legs to prevent 'runs'.

Note
Over the years the metal used for making biscuit tins has become thinner and sometimes, with rough use, the seams come apart. If the Peg Tin is used by a group, check frequently for sharp edges.

A way of avoiding this problem is to use individual coffee tins (with polythene lids) for each colour. These

66

new peg tins still have the hand-eye coordination and colour matching features of the large tin, but they will need fewer pegs, and can double up as simple one-hole posting boxes. Paint the tins — outsides only — and perhaps six pegs to match each one. Cut a small circle in the centre of each polythene lid. Check for rough or sharp edges, and trim them off or rub with sandpaper. The children match the pegs to the tins, and at the end of playtime can post them into the correct tin.

Colour Blocks on a Tray

Long-lasting

The first version of this toy was made for Frances. She attended the hospital school where I then worked. She had many disabilities, including poor hand function, but could recognise colours and handle chunky objects. One day I felt the urge to spruce up a tray full of bricks which had seen long service and I thought of her. The shabby bricks had been one colour all over. It seemed a boring and time-consuming job simply to repaint them — all that waiting for the paint to dry! — so I decided to paint each face of a brick a different colour. Armed with my little pots of red, blue, green, yellow, black and white Humbrol enamel, I set to work. With so many faces to cover, the first ones were nearly dry by the time I reached the end of the line, and with care I could start on the next colour. Next day at school, the result was sensational! Frances, not normally keen to exert herself, was obviously delighted by this shiny new 'toy'. She soon discovered how to turn the bricks over to reveal a different colour. At first, she arranged the bricks with all one colour on the top. Then she tried turning them about until she made stripes. On other days we showed her how to alternate the colours as in a chess board, and how to copy sequences and patterns we sketched for her with felt pens on squared paper.

When the toy library building bricks have needed a face lift, I have made smaller sets which have proved very popular with the children. Nine blocks will usually fit nicely into a margarine box, and this saves making a tray.

Colour Threading

Quick

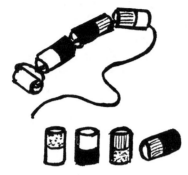

Turn to p. 180 and read about the conversion of cardboard till rolls into a threading toy. These tough rolls can also be used for more thought-provoking threading — not only must the roll end up on the threader, but it must match its neighbour by colour. This can make an interesting occupation for a quick-thinking child with less than perfect hand control.

Collect at least a dozen till rolls from your friendly supermarket checkout. Each half of a roll must be painted a different colour, say red and green for one, green and orange for the next, then orange and black .... and so on. After painting, the reels are protected with a coat of polyurethane varnish. When they are finished they are stored in a box. The child is provided with a threader. (Polypropylene washing line *without* a wire core.) She threads the first roll and is shown that the top colour is, say, red. She must now rootle in the box to find another roll with red on it, and add that to the threader so that the red halves touch. Now there will be a new top colour to search for. She continues this way, matching the colours domino fashion, until the threader is full.

Colour Matching Mat

Long-lasting

One day a friendly shopkeeper offered me an unwanted swatch of plain material in many colours. This was an offer I could not refuse!

I decided to make a colour matching activity for a group of older children, who were already familiar with the colours of the rainbow. I took the swatch apart, and picked out the samples of brown, navy blue, pink, grey, purple and turquoise. These were stitched together to make a mat. It was lined to make it machine washable. To prevent the colours from clashing too badly, strips of black bias binding were sewn over each seam. Next I collected various objects to match the colours on the mat. At first, this seemed a somewhat daunting task but, once the search had begun, one thing led to another. Take brown for instance, I soon found a felt pen, a comb, a plastic button, a leather button and a shoelace. Then I started to 'think brown', and added a fir cone, a conker, a bow of brown ribbon and an (empty!) tin of shoe polish. The same collecting process was repeated for all the other colours. If I was really stuck, I made a small toy—a ball or maybe a little grey mouse—of felt, or dressed an instant doll (p. 202) in the required colour. The mat and all the goodies were stored in a large polythene box with a lid.

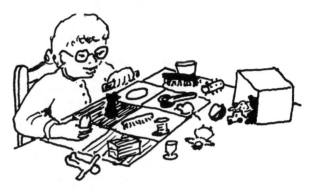

In play, the mat was spread out on the table, and each child was allotted a colour. The box was held high so that the children could not peep in, and they took it in turns to have a lucky dip. Each object was placed on the appropriate colour on the mat. Everyone watched intently, and made sure the right objects landed up on *their* patch. All this led to much animated conversation and frequent repetition of the colour names as the objects were identified and discussed. Previously, all the children's colour matching activities had been an exact match. Through this one, they began to realise, probably for the first time, that each colour could come in many shades.

The mat was also useful as an individual activity. A child could enjoy handling the real things at his own pace but, of course, the conversational opportunities were not the same.

Sometimes I found the mat constricting. Other groups of children might need primary colours or fewer choices. There was a simple solution to both problems. I painted squares of thick card in the colours I needed and protected them with clear, sticky-backed plastic. I put each card and all its bits and pieces in a bag made from net curtaining, which made it easy to see the colour inside. I kept them all together in a tough carrier bag. Now the organisation of the activity was easy. I chose the bags which were suitable for each group, gave out the cards and tipped all the coloured items into a box. The children formed the cards into a mat, then dipped in the box, matching the objects with the cards as before. At the end of the game each card and all its bits was returned to its bag, ready for next time.

If you are looking for a new colour matching activity the Colour Matching Mat is worth considering because:

- it is motivating and makes for variety and surprise;
- it uses three-dimensional objects which the children can handle;
- it is easy to change the objects or increase their number;
- as well as colours, other words can be practised — big and little, round and square, etc;
- it can be quickly adapted to individual requirements;
- if a few pieces go astray, they are easily replaced;
- best of all ... it is quick and simple to make.

Shake and Make

Long-lasting

Jackie Mills,
Hospital Play Specialist

This game is a favourite with the children on Jackie's ward. It could be equally successful in other group situations, or as a family game. All can take part on equal terms, and there need be no winners or losers. It also practises the skills of colour matching, counting up to six, and doing up press studs.

Jackie says the game was inspired by the Feely Caterpillar on p. 153. Shake and Make consists of a large number of little felt cushions which can be joined together with press studs. There must be six colours to correspond to the six sides of a die. Jackie chose red, blue, green, yellow, orange and black. The game also needs two dice; one with black spots from one to six, and the other with single coloured spots to correspond to the colours of the cushions.

Each child takes his turn at throwing both dice, then collects the cushions as directed. Supposing the dice show three spots and the colour red, the player helps himself to three red cushions and joins them together with the press studs. Next turn he might add two blue, then five green, etc., until all the cushions are used up.

For an individual activity, forget about the dice and just use the cushions for colour matching or making patterns. They can be joined together as a string of all one colour, or a sequence of colours can be repeated to make a pattern. The children in the hospital ward discovered another possibility. A string of cushions could be sent rolling down the long hospital corridor in a most satisfactory way!

Materials
- Felt in six colours.
- Polyester fibre for the stuffing.
- Press studs, or Velcro for younger and less able children.
- Two dice, numbered and coloured. Either use plastic ones — check that the colours match the colours of the felt — or make your own from cubes of plastic foam, covered with white material and decorated with the appropriate felt spots. On a number die, the opposite sides always add up to seven.
- A container for all the pieces.

Note
Blank plastic dice that you can mark yourself are available from Hope Education, page 4.

Method
To make a satisfactory game for four players you need *at least* ten cushions (twenty circles) in each colour. Cut the circles about 6 cm ($2\frac{1}{2}''$) in diameter. Use the foot of a wine glass or the base of a bottle for a template. Take two circles of one colour and tack them together, leaving a small opening for inserting the stuffing. Push in a small ball of polyester fibre, about the size of a ping-pong ball, and close the gap. Sew neatly all round the edge of the cushion — zigzag stitch on the machine, or oversew or blanket stitch by hand. Sew one half of a press stud to each side of the cushion, or use Velcro spots.

See also
The King of the Castle lost his Hat, p. 94.

TABLETOP MATCHING GAMES

When a child can pick out two identical pictures from a pile of jumbled-up pairs, she is ready to move on to one of the simpler games of picture-matching dominoes and lottos. These games call for accurate observation and an ability to wait your turn. They are also an excellent way of reinforcing the meaning of known words, and adding new ones to a child's vocabulary.

Dominoes

There are plenty of domino games in the toy shops, but they are so easy to make at home, and can be produced in so many ways, that it seems a shame not to have a go! Homemade ones can add variety to the commercial ones and, perhaps, make the game possible for children who cannot manage those on sale. For some ideas you will find Tactile Dominoes on (p. 209), Button Dominoes (p. 210) and some more made specially for children with a visual handicap on (p. 211). Turn to p. 65 for colour dominoes children can easily make for themselves. Very satisfactory picture dominoes can be made for older children with severe learning difficulties by using two identical mail order catalogues. Pick out the pictures of kettles, bicycles .... what you will. Cut out rectangles of card of a suitable size to take two pictures. Leave the first half of one rectangle blank, then add one of the pictures of a pair. Start the next rectangle with the twin picture, and finish it with the first picture of the next pair. Complete the set in this way. The last rectangle will end with a blank.

Picture Lottos

Lotto games consist of a set of base boards with pictures printed on them, and another set of the same pictures printed on small cards which, in play, are matched to those on the base boards. Usually all the little cards are shuffled up, then placed in a pile in the middle of the table. The children take it in turns to turn up the top picture. If they need it for their base board they keep it. If not, it is returned to the bottom of the pile. The game takes quite a long time to play by this method. For young children, or those with a short attention span, I change the rules a little! Everyone has a base board, but the method of distributing the small cards can vary according to the needs of the children playing. Perhaps they have very little, or no, speech, yet know the names of many objects. A leader who has no difficulty with words is appointed. (This is usually an adult.) The leader turns up the first card, says the name of the object on it, and if nobody recognises the word, shows the picture to the children. The one who needs it, claims it, and places it on top of the corresponding picture on her base board. The game continues until all the pictures on every base board are covered.

Young children with verbal ability like to play this way. The base boards are distributed and the small cards placed in the centre. One child picks a card, keeps the picture secret, but names the object on the card. The child who needs it, claims it. Taking turns in rotation, the next child turns up a card and, if lucky, it may be a picture she wants, so she can keep it. If not, she must give it away. If the game is played competitively, the child owning the first complete base board is the winner. Bingo!

Bought Lottos may not be suitable for young children with learning difficulties. The pictures are often too complicated, the pieces too numerous, and the time it takes to finish the game is likely to be too long for children with a short attention span. By the time they are mature enough to manage bought lottos, the pictures may be uninteresting to them and unsuitable for their age. The solution to all these problems is to make your own — a tailormade version.

A First Lotto

Long-lasting

This simple game is really just picture matching made into a group activity, but it helps children to understand the new idea of matching the pictures to a base board, and as it is a group game they have to wait for their turn. It is patently clear when they match the pictures correctly, and the eyes of every child will be following the matching process to make sure each player gets it right!

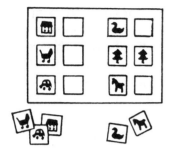

Materials

- Cardboard for the base boards and matching cards. (I used the fronts and backs of soap powder packets for my first set.)
- Pictures. Draw these yourself, (tracing off the second picture to make sure it matches) or use templates, or cut suitable pictures from gift wrapping paper, or buy a pack of Picture Identification Labels from NES Arnold, p. 4.
- PVA adhesive: craft knife and metal ruler for cutting the cardboard.
- Clear sticky-backed plastic for protecting the finished cards. (From large stationers or educational suppliers.)
- A container for all the pieces.

Method

First collect the pictures. The Picture Identification Labels mentioned above save a lot of effort and give a professional-looking result. They have an adhesive backing dispensing with the need for PVA adhesive. The size and number of pictures on the base board will, of course, determine its dimensions. Look at the illustration and arrange your pairs of pictures the same way. You may need more, or longer columns for your game. Rule up your base board in columns of pairs of squares (or rectangles) leaving a gap between each column. Stick one picture from each pair onto the base board. Stick the other to the small card which will, in play, be placed next to its partner on the base board. Wait until the adhesive is thoroughly dry, then cover all the pieces with clear sticky-backed plastic.

A Silhouette Shapes Lotto

Quick

This is a game that comes in useful when an activity for children of mixed ability is needed. Imagine the following situation. The crèche at the toy library had been busy all morning but, with only half an hour to go before closing time, just four children remained. They were an interesting little bunch. Jason, a mathematical wizard for his age, used words like 'conical' and 'rectangular' appropriately in his conversations, and was probably heading for a career in nuclear physics! Mary was shy and quiet, preferring to play alongside other children rather than with them. Peter, the youngest, had Down's Syndrome and was doing well. His latest achievement was to put the circle, square and triangle in the form board entirely on his own. Emma could now manage any game suitable for an average four-year-old, thanks to her new contact lenses. The crèche helpers had one eye on the clock and were thinking of all the clearing-up jobs ahead of them. One agreed to take the children in a corner, and try out the newly made Shapes Lotto, leaving the other helpers free to put the room to rights.

The children were interested in the new box, and Peter, as the youngest, was given the honour of removing the lid. Inside was a set of base boards, marked out in squares. Each square contained the silhouette of a geometrical shape. Some were simple, e.g. a square, others were more complicated, like a parallelogram or a tetrahedron. Under the base boards was a bag full of brightly coloured thick cardboard shapes which corresponded to the silhouettes. Before now, the children had always played Lotto games where pictures were matched. This time they must look carefully to make sure each black shape was properly covered. After a quick trial run, they soon discovered an oval was not the same as a circle, and a rectangle would not cover a square.

The game had eight base boards. The helper shared them round. Peter was given the one with the simple shapes he knew so well. Emma had two boards, placed at a comfortable distance for her to see easily. Jason was given the most complicated shapes and Mary and the helper looked after the rest. Each player dipped into the shapes bag in turn. The piece taken out was discussed and given to the one who needed it for their board. Anyone might be the 'first winner', but the game was not over until all the boards were complete.

This game can appeal to bright children like Jason because it is self corrective. For slow learners, or children with a visual impairment, it is a winner. Covering a black shape with a coloured one makes it obvious which shapes still have to be covered, and the board when filled looks satisfyingly colourful and complete.

Leafy Lotto

Long-lasting

This game makes use of real leaves from trees or plants, and makes a pleasant alternative to matching pictures or geometric shapes. It is particularly suitable for older children with learning difficulties.

Ideally the children help to collect the leaves. That in itself is a 'looking' challenge. It is surprisingly difficult to find a pair of leaves which are identical in every respect.

The game requires the usual base boards and small matching cards, plus as many pairs of leaves as possible. Press the leaves between blotting paper in a flower press or under a heavy pile of books. Leave them for a few days until they are dry and flat. With a little dab of PVA adhesive mount one leaf from each pair on a base board and the matching one on a small card. Protect all the cards with clear sticky-backed plastic.

Number Lotto

Long-lasting

This is a game for children who are already good at picture lottos. It will help them to recognise numbers up to thirty. It is made in the same way as the lottos above, but numbers from wall calendars take the place of pictures or shapes.

Tear off two calendar months. This will give you two sets of numbers from 1 to 30 (discard 31). To make a game for three players, measure the size of the number squares, then rule three base boards with ten squares on each line, corresponding in size to the number squares. In pencil, lightly indicate the numbers in the squares—1–10 on the top row, 11–20 in the middle, and 21–30 at the bottom. Cut up one of the calendar months and share the numbers among the base boards so that each card has two rows with three numbers on it, and one with four. (The line with four will be in a different position on each card.) Stick them down in their appropriate places and rub out the pencil lines in the unoccupied squares. Mount the other sheet of numbers on card, and cut them out when the glue is dry. Protect all the pieces with clear sticky-backed plastic and find a box to keep them in.

To Play

The caller has all the numbers in a box, face downwards,

76

and muddles them up. The players each have a base board. The caller picks out a number at random and calls out its name. If he does not know it, he shows it to the other players and hopefully they can prompt him! The number is matched to the correct place on a player's base board and all watch to make sure he gets it right. The game continues as the caller picks out all the other numbers one by one. We play non-competitively, and the game is not over until all the cards are filled.

FINGER PUPPETS

Instant

To make a finger puppet in a jiffy simply draw a little face on the front of a finger, yours or a child's, and wrap a handkerchief or tissue round it. It is immediately dressed in a hood and cloak! Keep this rudimentary clothing in place with a rubber band.

Very Quick

If you have an old pair of fabric gloves, cut off the best fingers and embellish them as suits your fancy, or as play dictates. Put your finger inside the potential puppet. This makes it easier to work on. Draw the eyes and mouth with felt pens, or if these will not show up well, indicate them with a few stitches. Stick on some wool or fur fabric 'hair' (PVA adhesive). Add some felt clothes, stitched or stuck, or use layers of lampshade trimming for a 1920s dress!

Quick

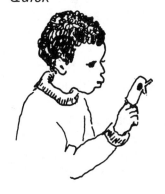

Now we come to a toy for knitters to make. The basic pattern is worked in stocking stitch. It can be made from odd scraps of wool, and the knitting part can be completed in less than twenty minutes! This makes it an excellent project for children who are just learning to knit. The puppet is finished before boredom sets in, and, if the body is knitted in stripes, it will appear to grow even more quickly.

Here is the basic pattern for an adult's finger. I suggest you follow it and try it for size. Then subtract a few stitches and knit a few less rows to make one

77

to fit a child. The finished puppet's body should cover the tip and at least the first joint of the finger. If it is too short and wide, it is likely to fall off, if too long and narrow, it is a struggle to fit it on.

Materials and Method

Use Double Knitting (DK) wool and size $3\frac{3}{4}$ (9) or $3\frac{1}{4}$ (10) needles. (With thinner wool use finer needles and cast on a few more stitches.)

Cast on 14 sts.

Knit two rows plain.

Knit 12 rows stocking stitch for the body. (One row plain, one row purl.)

Knit 10 rows stocking stitch for the head. (This will be a different colour if you are making a person.)

Break off a long length of wool and thread it through the stitches. Slide the stitches off the needle, draw the wool up tightly and sew the sides together. Your puppet now looks like the finger of a glove.

Make the head by pushing a small ball of polyester fibre into the tip. Bind with wool, just below the head. This will keep the filling in place and make a neck.

Now all your puppet needs is some individuality. The easiest character to make is a little bird. Just give your puppet two black french knot eyes, and a felt beak in a contrasting colour.

Finger puppets make splendid small presents, and any Mum, Auntie or Grandmother who makes a few to keep by for an emergency will bless the day she had such forethought! They are great for long journeys, as a little reward or as a consolation in a crisis. Margaret Hutchings, in her book *Making and Using Finger Puppets* describes how she uses them as a time-span indicator. She makes a little chest of drawers out of matchboxes. If a child is going to hospital for three days, her chest will have three drawers. One will contain a finger puppet, and another will be added the following day. When the chest is full it is 'Home Time!'

One of the highlights of the play sessions at our toy library at Kingston-upon-Thames is Music Time. The children and their Mums and Dads gather in a semi-circle round the piano to join in the action songs and finger plays. It is noticeable that the ones which include finger puppets hold the children's attention best. Their hand movements are larger and freer, and even the shy ones will join in. When the ritual of giving them out begins, the chosen child carries round the bag. It is obvious from the delight on the children's faces that they consider the best part of the session is about to begin. The puppets have an educational value too. We discuss the colours, count them, help each other put them on and sometimes swap. We have three favourite jingles that involve finger puppets and we ring the changes between them. 'Two Little Dickey Birds' is top favourite, closely followed by 'Two Grand Ladies'. When older children who are learning to count attend the session, we include 'Five Little Ducks'.

Two Little Dickey Birds

Knit another bird and you are ready to play 'Two Little Dickey Birds'. Here is the rhyme and the actions that go with it:

Two little dickey birds sitting on a wall, (Let puppets peep over the back of a chair or edge of the table.)
One named Peter, (Hold him up high)
The other named Paul. (Hold him up too)
Fly away Peter, (Hide him behind your back)
Fly away Paul, (Hide him too)
Come back Peter, (Bring him out from behind your back)
Come back Paul. (Bring him out too)

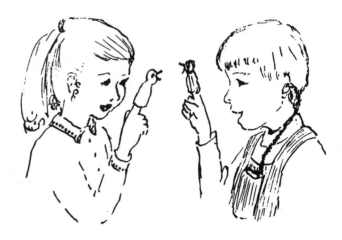

Two Grand Ladies

For the 'Two Grand Ladies', knit two puppets, changing to a head colour after the twelve rows stocking stitch. Make the ladies as grand as possible by adding wool hair, a felt hat with a feather in it, a satin cloak embellished with sequins .... let your imagination run riot! This is their rhyme:

Two grand ladies met in the lane, (Have the puppets on your index fingers, hold them apart and gradually bring them together)
Bowed most politely, bowed once again. (Make your fingers match the words and bow to each other)
'How do you do?' (One finger bows)
'How do you do?' (The other bows)
And 'How do you do?' again. (Both bow)

Five Little Ducks

Knit the basic pattern five times in yellow, add black eyes and orange bills and you have the five little ducks that went swimming. Make the Mother Duck as a snapper, using the pattern suggested below. Here is the rhyme for them:

Five little ducks went swimming one day,
Over the pond and far away. (Wear a duck on the fingers of one hand and make them 'swim' across the pond)
Mother Duck said 'Quack, quack, quack', (Use snapper puppet with the other hand, in time to the words)
And FOUR little ducks came swimming back. (Remove one puppet or bend your finger down)

Four little ducks were swimming one day etc.
Repeat until....
NO little ducks came swimming back.

Last verse....
Mother Duck went swimming one day,
Over the pond and far away.
Mother Duck said 'Quack, quack, quack',
And FIVE little ducks came swimming back.

Mother Duck Snapper Puppet

Quick

Mary Hurst,

Mary's snapper puppet is worked in wool over plastic canvas. Basically, it is made from three squares. The face and bottom jaw squares are extended to make the bill (*see diagram*.) When the three pieces are assembled, the back of the head acts as a spring, keeping the bill closed. Pinch the cheeks at the appropriate moment, and the puppet opens its bill to say 'Quack' on cue!

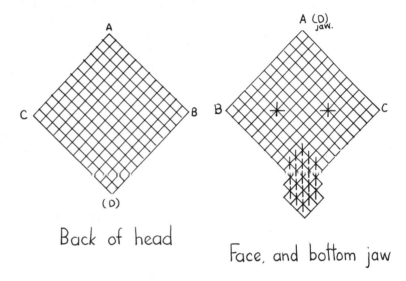

Back of head

Face, and bottom jaw

Materials
- Seven mesh plastic canvas (from a craft shop). This has eight bars — seven holes — to the inch.
- Wool — tapestry or DK used double — white for the head, yellow for the bill, black for the eyes.
- A tapestry needle. This has a large eye and a blunt point.

Method
Cut out a square of canvas for the back of the head. Make it 13 bars each way (12 holes).

Before cutting out the face and bottom jaw as in the diagram, I find it helpful to run a tacking stitch diagonally from point A through the middle of the bill to the tip. It is important that the tip of the bill lines up with point A. Count the bars carefully. It is very easy to snip an extra bar and make the bill too narrow. The cutting out is completed. Now for the stitching.

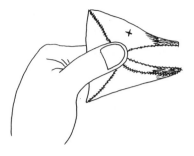

Cover the back of the head first, using tapestry stitch. Next, cover the face, as in the diagram, making the bill yellow and adding the eyes. These *must* be done at this stage. It is impossible to add them once the puppet is assembled. Then cover the bottom jaw the same way, but omitting the eyes of course! Finally, join all the pieces together by oversewing the appropriate edges. i.e. join AB on the face to AB on the back piece, and AC to AC. Make extra stitches at A to ensure the point is covered. Oversew the bottom jaw to the back by joining DB to DB and DC to DC.

In yellow, oversew all the way round the edges of the duck's bill. Now squeeze her cheeks to make her open her bill and appear to quack.

Snowman and Guardsman Finger Puppets

It is possible that you have now become addicted to knitting finger puppets! I guess you will think of many more characters to make. Here are two suggestions to start you off:

For a snowman, knit the puppet in white, add a black felt hat, features and a brightly coloured scarf.

To make a guardsman, start to knit in black for his trousers, change to red for his tunic, give him a pink face and top him with a black busby. Give him features and a wool chin strap. Add gold french knot buttons to his tunic and a felt belt.

Finger Puppets with Arms

Quick

These little puppets are very popular with the children who attend our toy library. Some are encouraged by their Speech Therapists to select, from a basketful, the characters they like best. We are told the puppets often lead to animated conversations. If the characters are knitted for an individual child, they can be made to represent various members of the family by giving them identifying characteristics — perhaps a bun and glasses for grandma, and a bald head for grandpa and so on.

Materials
Needles and scraps of wool, including a flesh colour, as for the finger puppets above.

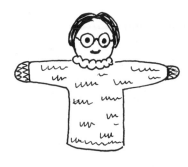

Method

The front and back are identical. They are knitted separately, then partly stitched together so that the hands can be added.

Here is the pattern. Knit it twice.

Cast on 8 st.
K 2 rows plain. K 12 rows stocking stitch.
The Arms. Cast on 4 st. K into the back of the first 5 st., then K to the end of the row.
Cast on 4 st. P into the back of the first 5, then P to the end of the row. (16 st.)
K 1 row.
P 1 row.
Cast off 6 st. (to make the shoulders). K to the end of the row.
Cast off 6 st. P to end of the row. (4 st.)
The Head. Break off the body colour and tie in the flesh colour.
K into the front and back of the first st., K 2. K into the front and back of the last st. (6 st.)
P 1 row.
Increase 1 st. at the beginning and end of the next row. (8 st.)
P 1 row.
Work 4 rows stocking stitch.
K 2 tog. at both ends of the next row. (6 st.)
P 1 row.
K 2 tog. at both ends of the next row. Break off wool and thread through the remaining 4 st. Do not cut it off. It is needed for sewing the sides of the head together.

With right sides together, join the front and back from the top of the head to the end of the arms. Use matching wool. Now add the *Hands.* Using flesh colour, pick up nine stitches across the end of a sleeve.

K 4 rows of stocking stitch. Break off wool. Thread through the stitches, draw up and stitch together the sides of the hand. Repeat the process for the other hand.

Complete the joining up.

Stuff the head with a small ball of polyester fibre and tie round the neck.

Bring your puppet to life by adding features, hair,

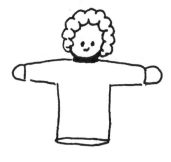

and extra adornments—buttons made from french knots, a lace collar, or perhaps a hat?

The body of the standard puppet lends itself to variations. The body can be knitted in two colours to represent jeans and a jersey, fabric clothes can be added—even 'props' like a tiny duster can be stitched to one hand, or a pom-pom ball tucked under a child puppet's arm. To make a baby, simply reduce the pattern by casting on less stitches (say 6) and working fewer rows.

Glove Puppets

Quick

Bought glove puppets are often too large and heavy for small hands, but it is easy for anyone handy with a needle to make one the right size.

First cut out a paper pattern. Place the child's hand on a piece of paper with the fingers and thumb in the position they will be when working the puppet. Most children like to use their thumb for one arm, their index finger for the neck and their middle finger for the other arm. The ring and little fingers are tucked into the palm. A few children prefer to use two fingers to work the head and two fingers for the arm not filled with the thumb. Draw round the child's hand in his chosen position, making a very generous seam allowance. Cut out the puppet in double material and tack round the seams. Try it for size before stitching properly, then decorate according to character. A slit up the back of the puppet's dress can make it much easier for some children to put their fingers in the right places.

Stitch two metal buttons to the hands of a glove puppet and it can play the 'cymbals'! A Physiotherapist found this idea useful when she was working with a child whose hands had been badly burnt. Wearing the puppet, the child was encouraged to make the cymbals clash in time to music, so bringing her finger and thumb together, and unwittingly performing her exercises!

MAKING THE MOST OF JIGSAWS

Some children never really take to jigsaws. This is a pity because they are such a good way of encouraging the careful observation of shape and colour. They can also be fun, and a rewarding and peaceful occupation for a child who must sometimes play alone. Perhaps the dislike started when a well-meaning adult tipped a box of pieces onto the table and expected the child to make that bewildering muddle into a picture. Many children in this situation will avoid criticism and failure by refusing to have anything to do with the puzzle, so it is important to choose a first one that the child can manage with confidence.

Inset puzzles

The best puzzles for beginners are inset puzzles. A simple picture is painted on plywood, and the individual shapes that make up the scene are cut out in one piece. Perhaps a person, a tree, a car and a house are removed. The picture now has gaps where the shapes should fit It is mounted on a hardboard backing (to prevent the pieces from falling through) and the child must fit the pieces in their rightful places and so complete the picture. The inset pieces on this type of puzzle are usually fitted with little knobs to make them easier to remove from the picture. If these knobs are too small for your child to handle, turn to p. 20 for some alternative means of removing pieces.

A Vinyl Tile Shapes Inset Puzzle

Quickly made and Long-lasting

This inset puzzle is useful for older children with severe learning difficulties. It also makes a change for younger ones who have become bored with their plywood inset puzzles (through long association!), but who still need practise in assembling a puzzle at this level of difficulty.

Vinyl tiles are produced in attractive colours and designs, and are easy for an adult to cut with a craft knife. A few are often left over from a DIY flooring job.

Suppose you want a puzzle consisting of only a circle and a square. A saucer might make a suitable template for the circle, and perhaps a tea caddy or other handy tin would do for the square. When the child can replace these shapes with confidence, try cutting them in half. Now two semicircles or two triangles (or rectangles) must be fitted into the spaces. A variety of smaller shapes can be made by using the pieces from a shapes sorter as templates. It may be easy to make a shape fit its hole but, if the pattern is also to match, it may be necessary to turn the shape about, and that will call for concentrated looking.

Non-inset puzzles

Now for some simple 'free standing' jigsaws, which can bridge the gap between inset puzzles and interlocking ones.

Christmas Card Jigsaws

Instant

These puzzles can be made in a flash from old Christmas Cards, so they can come in handy as a little diversion when a dull day needs cheering up. They are ephemeral toys so can be regarded as 'disposables'. This makes them particularly suitable for children with infectious complaints. They can also be useful to pop in your bag if you are travelling or facing a long wait.

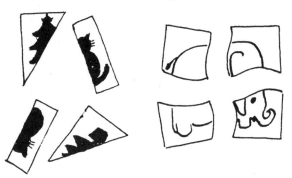

To make this simple puzzle easier to handle and more robust, glue the front of the card to the back before you cut it into two or more pieces. The task is more challenging if two cards with distinctive pictures — perhaps a cat and a fir tree — are cut up and the pieces muddled together. The child must first sort them out before assembling each puzzle.

Box Puzzles

Quick

Freda Kim,
Lekotek Korea,
Seoul

From the newsletter of Lekotek (Toy Library) Korea comes an excellent suggestion for using the strong cardboard boxes that package some toys, and recycling them to make simple jigsaws. Each box displays a colourful picture of the toy inside. This will be a familiar plaything to the child, so she will recognise its shape in the picture and should be able to complete the puzzle once she has understood the idea of fitting all the pieces together. All that needs to be done is to trim the picture with a craft knife (adults only!), then cut it into a few bold pieces.

Matchbox Puzzles from South America

Quick

Nylsa de Cunha,
Teacher,
Brazil

Nylsa is a teacher of children with special needs, and organises the Brazilian Association of Toy Libraries. She has the enviable skill of being able to create really useful 'teaching' toys from throw-away materials. Her lovely matchbox puzzles prove the point!

These puzzles are a novelty for all children, but are particularly suitable for those who have difficulty in handling the pieces of an ordinary jigsaw. The matchboxes are chunky, light and easy to grip, and can be manoeuvred with a 'Unicorn' head pointer or fist.

Collect, say, four matchboxes. (More for a more difficult puzzle.) To give them extra strength, stuff the tray of each box with a paper tissue. Return the tray to the box and wrap insulating tape (used by electricians) round the edges. This serves two functions: it keeps the drawers in place (and prevents the children from opening them) and, more importantly, covers the abrasive sides.

Hold the matchboxes together with masking tape, then stick a picture on each face. When the glue is dry,

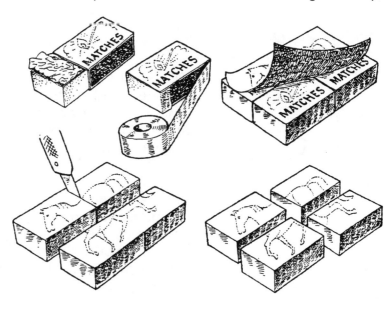

carefully separate the matchboxes by cutting between them with a craft knife.

I have tried out this idea and can vouch for its popularity. I used just four boxes and grouped them as in the illustration. On one side I pasted a horse and on the reverse side I stuck a picture of a tall giraffe. This meant the boxes had to be arranged a different way to complete each puzzle and the children had to look extra carefully at the picture to see how the parts joined up.

My matchbox puzzle had its greatest moment of glory when it was successfully put together by a little girl with cerebral palsy. The most controllable part of her body was her head. With the help of her Unicorn head pointer and a baking tray fixed to the table with Blu-tac, she was able to push the chunky boxes against the top edge of the tray, then slide them into the corner in the right order to complete the picture.

Wooden Push Together Puzzles

Long-lasting

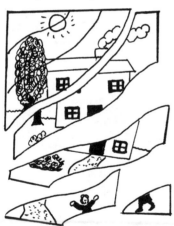

Imagine you have painted a picture on plywood and have divided it in two by cutting a wavy line down the middle. Before you is the simplest possible push together puzzle. If you are fortunate enough to have the use of a band saw or an electric jigsaw, you are in a position to make these puzzles by the dozen. Each picture can be cut into as many pieces as appropriate for the child in question just by cutting more wiggly lines.

This type of puzzle is specially suitable for children with poor hand control because the shapes do not have to be lifted, but are simply pushed together. One has been assembled by a child with her hands heavily bandaged, and another used his feet.

For such special needs, the pieces need to be confined on a tray with a lip—a biscuit baking tray anchored to the working surface with Sticky Fixers or Blu-tac is a good choice. The child can push the first piece of the puzzle into a corner and then line up all the other pieces in order alongside it. When using a baking tray as a working surface, it may be helpful to apply small pieces of magnetic tape (p. 3) to the backs of the puzzle pieces. This slows down the sliding action and makes it easier to line up the pieces accurately.

Interlocking jigsaws

The next stage in jigsaw puzzling is to assemble one with interlocking pieces. Firstly, the child must realise that the separate shapes can be linked together to make a picture. The simplest way of explaining this is to show him slowly how it is done! Make the puzzle, but hand him the final piece — the right way round — to fit in the last hole. The next time the puzzle is made, he puts in the final piece and perhaps one of the corners.... and so on, always finishing the picture. He will soon know what he is aiming at, and will finally be ready to make the whole puzzle from scratch. Explaining the puzzle in this way is an example of 'backward chaining'.

Two-Piece Jigsaws

Long-lasting

In the early days of Kingston Toy Library (before I had learnt the 'backward chaining' technique described above), I was watching a small child trying to put together a simple interlocking jigsaw. We had first shown him the completed puzzle, and he had helped us to take it apart. He realised he must put the pieces together again but, without looking at the colour clues, try as he might, he could not force the pieces to fit. He had the right idea, but was looking at the shape and disregarding the picture. This cross and frustrated little boy started me thinking. Why not make two-piece puzzles which must be matched by colour?

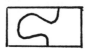 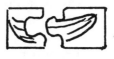

The first set was made in the local Occupational Therapy workshop. It consisted of eight rectangles of chunky plywood, each one painted a different colour and cut across the centre with a wiggly line to create two interlocking pieces. In play, all the puzzles were taken apart and the pieces muddled up. (We say 'Stir the pudding' for this operation!) The children were eager to find two pieces the same colour and put them together again.

Audrey Stevenson, a toy designer and friend of the toy library, turned this simple idea into a really good toy by painting a picture on the reverse side of each puzzle, e.g. one side yellow, and on the flip side a banana — or green on one side and a tree on the reverse. With all this colour and picture matching, the children not only became adept at linking together interlocking pieces, but also at *looking* at the pictures and pairing the pieces before joining them together.

Two other sets of these simple jigsaws were made for children with specific play problems. The first was for a bright little girl of two-and-a-half who had brittle bones. Her hands were small and her reach limited, so the pieces for her puzzles were tiny, and cut from three-ply. Instead of making all the puzzles rectangular, other geometric shapes were introduced — circle, triangle, square, hexagon — and these were cut into two or more pieces. Pictures illustrating nursery rhymes were painted on one side and patterns adorned the reverse of each puzzle. The second set was made for a five-year-old with very poor hand control. His teacher made him a special set of two-piece puzzles. She bought several picture postcards, mounted them on block board (which is thick and fairly light). Interlocking pieces were not for this child, so she divided each picture with a wavy line. She would muddle the pieces from two or three puzzles and put them in front of him. With some persistent effort the little boy could sort out the pairs, push them in order against the lip of his tray and reconstitute the pictures.

Edge Jigsaws

Long-lasting

I made my first edge jigsaw soon after I learnt about 'backward chaining'. It seemed a waste of time to cut out all the pieces if I was to be the one to put most of them together again! I found it particularly useful when working with older children with severe learning difficulties.

To them it was intriguing, and they were usually motivated to sit at it until the picture was completed. With this type of puzzle the maker can follow the clues of colour and shape given by the bulk of the picture in the middle. He also learns that straight edges go on the outside.

Instead of cutting the whole puzzle, I simply cut

some pieces from the edge (as though taking bites out of it!), leaving the whole of the centre intact. I sand-papered all the pieces, replaced them, and painted a picture suitable for older children. In order to avoid waste, and to make two puzzles for the price of one, the reverse was decorated with a black and white design. Some children preferred this side to the picture!

LOOKING AROUND

Some instant suggestions

The next time morale is low because rain bespatters the window pane, turn the raindrops into a looking game and have races between them! When the weather cheers up and you are indoors by a sunny window, why not play with Jack-a-dandies? These are the brilliant reflections made by sunlight bouncing off a shiny object, and can easily be made to 'dance' on the ceiling. Small, unbreakable mirrors make splendid Jack-a-dandies, but any shiny surface will do, even a bowl of water. (Slightly ruffle the surface to make changing, delicate patterns.) Perhaps, when you were at school, you assumed an air of innocence as you reflected the sun off your knife and dazzled your friend! There is a knack in controlling a Jack-a-dandy — for a start the shiny object must face the sun. To direct the reflection in a certain direction calls for consider-able hand-eye coordination!

At night time, Torch Hee is a good game to play in the dark. Each player has a hand torch. One switches on and directs her beam over the walls and ceiling. The other player switches on and tries to impose her beam on the first one. When she succeeds, it is her turn to switch on first ... or just make up the rules as you go along.

Seeing Saunter

This is the kind of walk when time is of no consequence. So often this is not the case. Time presses and the ground must be covered as quickly as possible. Not so on a Seeing Saunter. The distance covered may only be to the end of the street but, on the way, there will have been time to examine the patterns on the drain covers, notice the designs in the brickwork of the houses, admire the gardens, find plants growing in unlikely places, read the numbers on the gates, even perhaps find some adventurous insects also out for a stroll. Whatever the child's environment may be, town, country or in between, for those who look, there are always fresh things to discover.

A String Ring

Adopt a scientific sampling technique. Make a 'string ring' and you have an unusual way of focusing your child's attention on one tiny patch of the world that surrounds him. Imagine you are both sitting on the grass. All you have to do is to mark out a small area with a circle of string and peer intently into it! Soon you both will notice not only the grass with its many shades of green, but also the plants and mosses, all contributing to the greenery. Look carefully, and you might see a worm throwing up a cast, or a tiny insect struggling through the jungle of leaves. Because the area under scrutiny is defined by the string ring, your child is less likely to be distracted by the wider view and some concentrated observation should result. What a pleasant way of 'learning to look'.

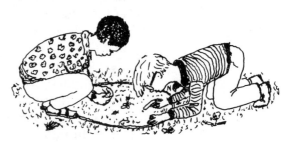

Shopping Search

Quick

Try this searching activity when next you visit the supermarket.

Susan's Mum invented 'Shopping Search'. Susan was a profoundly deaf little girl. Her mother was always looking for an opportunity to enlarge her vocabulary and help her associate words with objects. She made a collection of pictures of food. She found these in magazines, or on the tins and packets in her store cupboard. Each picture was mounted on card (possibly the backs of old Christmas cards), and the name of each item was written under its picture. Before each shopping expedition, she would show her shopping list to Susan who would then match the word on the list to the one under the picture. All the necessary pictures were taken to the supermarket, where Susan could search for the real thing among the shelves. This game is a winner. It can turn a sometimes stressful shopping expedition into an enjoyable experience packed full of learning! It is especially recommended for children with speech problems, slow learners, and the busy ones!

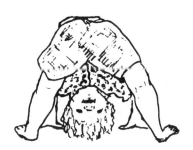

LOOKING AT THE WORLD A DIFFERENT WAY

Babies learning to walk soon discover they can look through their legs and have an entrancing view of an upside-down world. All children seem to like to play tricks with what they see. The following suggestions may encourage some interesting experiments:

- Peeping through fingers;
- Looking down a cardboard tube;
- Looking through coloured cellophane;
- Looking through homemade 'rose tinted spectacles' —frames from pipe cleaners, lenses from cellophane;
- Looking through a piece of paper with a hole in it;
- Playing with a mirror. A plastic baby mirror, available from toy shops, is double-sided and very robust;
- Holding up a mirror on a handle and seeing what is behind you;
- Using a magnifying glass (plastic ones are available from Opticians) or microscope;
- Looking through a telescope or pair of binoculars —either way round;
- Looking through a kaleidoscope to see the ever-changing patterns;
- Looking through an octoscope. This is similar to a kaleidoscope, but instead of producing patterns, it

reflects many times whatever it is pointed at. This could be a person's face, the view from the window, the child's hand, etc. Available from many toy shops, gift shops, etc.

GAMES WHICH ENCOURAGE CHILDREN TO LOOK

Peep–Bo

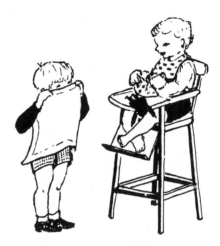

This old favourite has been enjoyed by babies since time immemorial. It is the element of anticipation and surprise that they find so delightful. A face, or a teddy, that pops up from behind the back of the arm chair — sometimes over the top, sometimes round the side — is sure to appeal to the baby's sense of humour.

The King of the Castle Lost His Hat

Everyone knows the time-honoured game of 'I spy with my little eye', where one player says the initial letter of an object, and the others must try to guess what he has spied. This game is excellent for encouraging a child to look around and notice things, but it is too difficult for children who have not yet learnt about letter sounds. The King of the Castle Lost His Hat only requires the child to be able to identify some colours. It can be made as simple as necessary. The leader thinks of an object in the room. It could be the carpet, or a cushion, or perhaps the ribbon in someone's hair. He then says the nonsense rhyme .....

The King of the Castle lost his hat,
Some say this, and some say that ....
But I say Mr Green..
(or Blue, or Red, etc. according to the colour of the object he has chosen.)

The other children must try to guess the 'Green' thing. The person who gets it right, takes over as leader for the next turn. As skill increases the colours can be made more difficult, e.g. 'Mr Black and Silver' might be the knob on the television set.

Getting it Wrong Again

Instant

Lorraine Crawford,
Speech Therapist

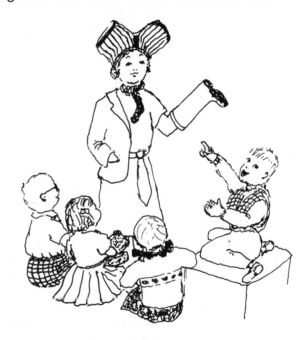

If you want to add a touch of hilarity to the day, try the game Lorraine sometimes uses. She has a box full of dressing-up clothes, and in front of a group of children with learning difficulties *she* chooses a garment and deliberately puts it on wrongly—back to front, upside-down, inside out, shoes on her hands, socks on her ears! There is no end to the possibilities, and you can imagine the concentrated looking, laughter and speech this game sparks off.

Kim's Game

Instant

This is a game requiring keen observation and a good memory. It can easily be adapted to meet the needs of children of varying ages and abilities. It is usually played as a group game, but works just as well with one child and an adult.

The Basic Game
Arrange some easily recognisable objects on a tray, e.g. a matchbox, cotton reel, thimble, button, pencil, etc. The number of the objects chosen will depend on the ability of the child. He then has time to look at all the objects, and memorise their position on the tray. He hides his eyes while one object is removed. When he opens them, he has another look at the tray and guesses which object is missing. Then it is his turn to remove an object for you to identify.

Variations
Instead of taking an object away, another can be added to the tray, or the position of two objects can be interchanged. Sometimes the child can help to collect the items for the tray, perhaps choosing only round shapes, or rectangular ones, or those of a certain colour. Because he has contributed to the collection, a child with a poor memory will have a better chance of identifying them.

The Limpet Shell Game

Instant — once a supply of shells have been collected

Paula Campbell, Parent

Paula's family was spending a holiday near a beach which was strewn with limpet shells. The shape and feel of these fascinated the children, and they spent a happy time collecting a vast hoard. At the end of the day, of course, they had to be taken home to be gloated over again.

As so often happens when there is a surfeit of one thing, someone comes up with a clever idea of making use of it. Paula thought of a quiet and peaceful game which riveted the children's attention on the shells and did wonders for their powers of observation!

Everyone sat around in a circle, and each person received the same number of limpet shells, say seven. The leader chose a shell from her collection and put it in the middle of the circle.

Everyone searched through their little pile to find the one which most closely resembled the leader's. Maybe it was nearly the same colour, or had an irregularity on one side, or was almost identical in size.

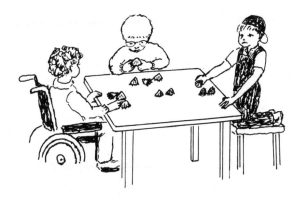

(Try finding two limpet shells *exactly* the same, and you will see their problem!) Finally, everyone made their choice and put their shell near the leader's. She then had the task of weeding them out, one by one, until only the shell she considered to be most like hers remained. The owner of that one glowed with pride and became the next leader.

If you don't have a supply of limpet shells handy, I guess the game would work just as well with stones or leaves.

Searching games

All searching games like 'Hunt the Thimble' or 'Hide and Seek' are good for encouraging children to look. A 'Treasure Hunt' usually meets with child approval too. This does not necessarily have to be planned in advance. Small children are content with a simple version where they are asked to find, for instance, a yellow flower, or a white stone, or maybe something square.

The Puzzle Game

Quick

(This game was developed from the Christmas Card Puzzles, p. 86.)

When our family was young and birthday parties were a regular festivity, this game was often used as a 'starter'. It kept the guests busy and happy until everyone had arrived and the fun could begin in earnest. It needed a little advance preparation, but always got the party off to a happy start. Plenty of Christmas Cards were cut into pieces. One piece of each puzzle was kept in a paper bag. All the other pieces were hidden somewhere in the room. The children took a piece from the bag, then had to search around to find the rest of the picture. Every time a picture was completed, the child received a small sweet to keep his strength up for the next search!

AIMING GAMES

Ball games are often the child's first experience of playing an organised game with someone else. While the play lasts, child and adult have each other's undivided attention, and both can find this very enjoyable.

Rolling games

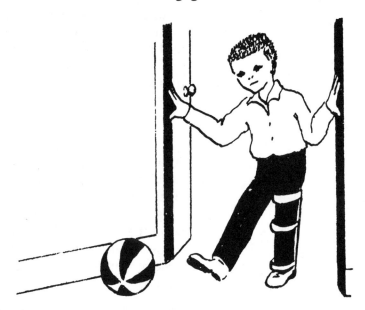

Playing Goal Keeper

Instant

This is a way of helping a child to keep his eye on the ball. He stands in a doorway. If he finds it difficult to balance while he kicks, he can use the door posts for support. The ball is rolled towards him, along the hall or landing. Make the distance as long as possible so that he has plenty of time to see the ball coming.

All ball games are excellent for encouraging children to look, and it is not hard to adapt ball play to meet the requirements of almost any child. When a baby can sit unsupported, he may be ready for the simplest of all ball games. Just aim for his hand and slowly roll a large and colourful ball across the floor towards it. When he 'catches' the ball, he will probably want to put it in his mouth and generally explore it. After a while, he will be willing to give it up for the joy of having it bowled to him again. Some children like to sit with their legs apart, forming a sort of harbour. This certainly makes it easier for them to field the ball. The next stage is for the child to return the ball to you. Already he is starting to learn a basic ball skill as he tries to aim in a certain direction. When he realises how difficult this is, I guess his sense of humour will come to the fore and he will have more fun deliberately mis-aiming and making you chase after the ball!

Throwing and catching games

At the early stages of teaching a child to throw and catch, there is a lot to be said for using beanbags instead of balls. Beanbags can be made any size, and any weight. They nestle into the hand nicely, are easy to grasp and they *do not roll away or bounce*.

Beanbags

Quick

Monica Taylor,
Normansfield Hospital

Monica made large cylindrical beanbags, filled with polystyrene packaging chips. These made a pleasant rustly sound when squeezed, and are harmless if they are badly aimed! Most people make beanbags about 10 × 15 cm (4 × 6″), and half fill them with rice or dried peas. Of course, these will not wash. (Anyone who has accidentally put one in the washing machine will have learnt that lesson the hard way!) I like to use fish grit, from a pet shop, as a filling. It is heavier than rice, and makes the beanbags easier for some children to control. As my bags are washable, it does not matter if they are kicked around the floor or accidentally left out in the rain. I make the covers from strong cotton. Sometimes our local scrap bank has a supply of offcuts of nylon sail cloth or kite material. This comes in brilliant colours and is extremely strong. It makes excellent covers. My favourite beanbags are made in terry towelling and are shaped like starfish. The irregular shape makes them attractive to look at and much easier to hold.

Aunt Sally

Quick

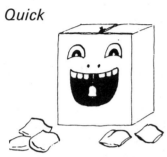

This throwing game is suitable for a group of children of mixed ages and ability. A handicapping system can be agreed upon. A large grocery carton has a cheerful face painted on one side. The mouth is cut away to make a large hole through which the beanbags can be thrown. A bell is suspended from the roof of the box, like a giant epiglottis. Every time a beanbag sails through the mouth, the bell rings to signal success!

Toss in the Bin

Instant

This game is even easier to organise. Put a grocery carton or waste paper basket on the floor. Let the child stand fairly close at first, and throw in the beanbags. As skill increases, he stands further away. This game also comes in handy at clearing up time. Play it with all the spilt Lego bricks!

Throw and Catch

Instant

Christine Cousins,
Educational Psychologist

This game is the reverse of the one above. In this case, *you* do the throwing, while the child receives your missiles in a cardboard carton. This needs to be held firmly in *both hands*. Throw in objects of different weights to land on the bottom with a satisfying thud.

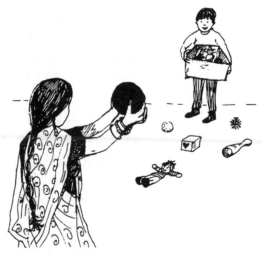

Another Target Game

Instant

Dr Roy McConkey

In one of his lectures, Dr McConkey, an expert on play for people with special needs, suggested an instant throwing game, packed full of activity. It can be played by two people, at any time, anywhere, for all it requires is a carrier bag and a modest supply of scrap paper. The paper is folded into paper darts, and one player hurls these into the carrier bag held open by the other. The bag man aims to catch as many darts as possible. Remembering the erratic flight of most paper darts, the catcher must *catch* the approaching missile and move nimbly to trap it in his bag.

THREE SOCK GAMES FOR LETTING OFF STEAM

The Comet Game

Instant

As a game for two or more older children, all this one requires is plenty of open space to run about in, and an old sock with a tennis ball, (or a tightly crunched up ball of newspaper) tied in the toe. The children stand a little way apart. One holds the sock by the leg, twirls it round, and at the right moment lets it go. It will fly through the air with the leg of the sock streaming out behind like the tail of a comet. The task for the other child is to try to catch the 'comet' by the tail.

Sock Fights

Instant — for two or more

Maureen McEvoy, Parent

This game bears a strong resemblance to the ever popular one of pillow fighting. The advantage of this one is that the 'biffer' is considerably smaller and, therefore, less likely to damage either players or property. To make a 'biffer', put a foam ball (or a handful of cottonwool balls) in the toe of a sock and tie a knot half way up the leg to keep the stuffing in place. Any rules must be clearly understood before battle commences. It is as well to encourage biffing only below shoulder height. The head area *must* be out of bounds if glasses are worn, and hits there should be heavily penalised — perhaps with a trip to the 'sin bin'?

Human Skittles

Instant Group Game

Human Skittles was invented for a group of teenagers with learning difficulties who were in residential care. It called for controlled activity, and soon became one

101

of their favourite games. It was played in the recreation room where the odd wild throw would do no damage. All it required was a quantity of odd socks (donated by the care staff, and topped up from time to time) and a box to keep them in. Each sock was rolled up into a ball. (A good activity for encouraging manual dexterity!) It did not matter if they became unrolled in flight — they were just less likely to reach the target. They could easily be re-rolled for the next go.

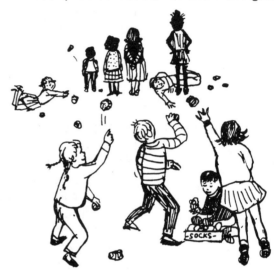

The players were divided into two groups, the 'skittles' and the 'throwers', who had to keep their distance by making sure their toes were behind the edge of the carpet. When a 'skittle' was hit, it had to topple to the ground, and when all were down the teams changed places. It usually took some time to reclaim all the socks. Plenty of bending and stretching needed for this job.

The game was noisy and lively, but also disciplined. The box of socks could not be raided until both teams were in place, and throwing had to wait until the umpire said the ritual 'One, two, three, GO!'

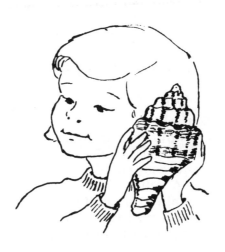

Making the most of HEARING

LEARNING TO LISTEN

It is nine o'clock and the children are arriving at nursery school. There is a cheerful hubbub as mitts are stuffed into pockets and hats and coats hung on the low pegs. From one classroom comes the sound of a tape recorder playing Mendelssohn's 'A Midsummer Night's Dream' Overture. The children in Miss Clarke's class hurry towards the sound, and sit quietly on the little chairs, listening to the fairy music. In the music, they hear the sound of a donkey braying. They giggle, enjoying Miss Clarke's little joke. Yesterday, Michael had brought Neddy, his cuddly donkey, to school. Everyone had admired and stroked this well-loved toy and learnt to bray. They listen to part of the music again, and everyone joins in with the eeyores. Miss Clarke tells them about a real donkey she knows, and they listen attentively to a story about his misdemeanours. Then they learn the nursery rhyme . . .

If I had a donkey and he wouldn't go
Do you think I'd wallop him? Oh no no!
I'd put him in a stable and keep him nice and warm,
The best little donkey that ever was born.

Today's big news is centred round the conch shell an uncle has given to one of the children. All have a turn at listening to the sound of the sea in the shell. Brian is bored at having to keep quiet while the others listen. He plays with his ear, and discovers he can make almost the same sound of the sea by cupping his hand over it. He tells the group about his discovery and they all try it for themselves. Mary runs to the junk box and puts a yoghurt pot over her ear, but the result is disappointing. Miss Clarke takes two tins from the junk box and with a skewer, makes a small hole in the bottom of each. She threads a long piece of string through the holes in the tins to join them together, and ties large knots on the ends, so that it will not pull out. With the string held taut between them, she shows two children how they can use the tins as a telephone — one speaking into his tin, while his friend listens at the other end. The children soon learn that they must keep the string really tight, but this inevitably becomes a tug-of-war. Miss Clarke saves the situation by asking her assistant to hold one end while she supports the other. Now the children need only to speak or listen and the crude telephone is working beautifully.

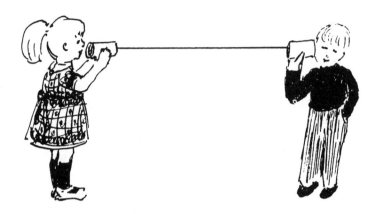

Michael and Mandy have gone to play in the music corner. Yesterday Michael discovered that if he chose the chime bars for *doh*, *ray*, and *me* he could play 'Mary Had a Little Lamb'. He had spent many minutes trying to perfect his performance, and now he wants to repeat his success. Brian comes over to investigate. He knows that if you push a strip of cardboard backwards and forwards under a chime bar, you can make the note 'wobble'. They play the nursery rhyme with a wide vibrato, and sing along in high pitched voices.

Mandy has noticed a long Slither Box (p. 115) which is new to the music corner. At first she tips the box this way and that, enjoying the feeling of the grit being transferred from one hand to the other, and the sharp slapping sound it makes as it reaches each end. Her arms begin to tire, and she tips the box more slowly, noticing the soft, shooshing noise she is now making. She has heard that sound before. Now she remembers. It was a stormy day at the seaside. Huge waves dashed against the promenade, and made that same shooshing noise as they sucked back the pebbles in the foamy undertow.

Sharon is sad today. She was slow to wake up and the day has turned out badly. She has crept beneath the branches of the weeping willow tree that grows

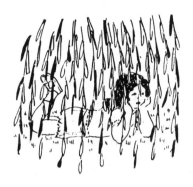

in a corner of the outside play area. She wants to find a private place where she can be alone and nurse her grievances. A slight breeze flutters the long, slender leaves on the dangling branches, making a very soft rustling sound. Sharon is absorbed in watching and listening, her troubles quite forgotten. The breeze dies away and the leaves hang limply. The soothing sound has stopped. She grasps a branch and shakes it vigorously, but the sound is not the same.

Time for lunch. The children have been playing in the band. They return their instruments to the rack. Soon everyone is washed and tidy, and ready for lunch. Before long the plates are empty, and some of the children help to stack them up. One has discovered that she can push her spoon over a plate in a certain way and produce an ear-splitting noise. She laughs at the instant reaction of the nursery nurse, and repeats the horrible sound twice more before the plate is swiftly removed!

After lunch comes rest time. Soon most of the children, used to the regular routine, are fast asleep. Martin is new to the nursery and he lies awake listening to the muted sounds from the other parts of the building. The clatter from the kitchen, laughter from the staff room, an ambulance hurrying by in the street, the sound of a child breathing heavily, the rustle of the page as the nursery nurse starts a new chapter in her book — he hears all these everyday sounds before he, too, falls asleep.

And so the day continues. So far, it has been a mixture of concentrated listening initiated by the adults, quiet times, noisy times and plenty of opportunities to play with sounds. These children have certainly been making the most of their hearing.

MAKING OPPORTUNITIES FOR ATTENTIVE LISTENING AT HOME

For young children

Consider the neighbours, and the rest of the family, but when the time is right, look around the kitchen

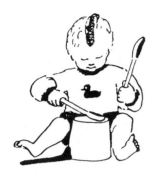

for some 'instant' percussion instruments. A wooden spoon and an upturned saucepan or biscuit tin will make a perfect drum. Two tough plastic egg cups can be banged together to make a noise like castanets, and an old spoon stirred round a wire sieve will make a gentle whirring sound . . . The child is sure to invent her own sounds. A three-year-old of my acquaintance illustrates this point. She had nearly finished eating her yoghurt. In her efforts to scrape up every bit, she was running her spoon round the bottom of the pot. This had ridges, like the spokes of a wheel. She found that drawing her spoon over these made a loud and distinctive sound quite capable of stopping the mealtime conversation.

Use a particular sound to anticipate a certain activity. In Victorian families a gong would summon everyone to the meal. In modern times the Ship's Bell rattle (p. 114) might serve the same purpose. Even a simple action, such as splashing your hand in the water before putting a child in the bath, will give him a sound clue of what is about to happen.

If you can remember to say 'Up you come' every time before picking baby up, the frequent repetition will help him to recognise the 'tune' of the phrase long before he can understand the words. The daily routine can be full of such noisy little incidents, and each will help a child to be more aware of his surroundings and add to his sense of security.

Speak and sing to your child as much as you can. Describe your actions as you care for him and go about your work. All babies need to listen for many months before they are ready to try to make the sounds of speech. Some children with special needs may need a very long listening time before they can sort out all the sounds that surround them. If they do not appear to respond, or if they are 'good' and content to lie quietly until the next meal, it is so easy to forget to keep up the chatter! Nursery rhymes and finger plays and jingles for body awareness like 'This little piggy went to market' can come to the rescue!

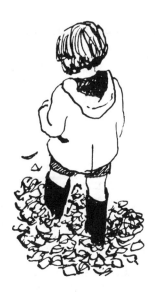

For older children

Try taking your child on a 'listening loiter'. Like the 'Seeing Saunter' on p. 91, the object of this particular walk is not to reach a destination, but to stop and listen at frequent intervals to all the sounds going on around. If you listen really hard, you will be surprised at the number you can identify in quite a short while. It is also fun for children to use the environment for making sounds — perhaps jumping on a drain cover, scuffing through the autumn leaves, dragging a stick along a wooden fence or across iron railings, blowing across a blade of grass held tightly between the thumbs — what a variety of sounds can be created by even these few activities.

Few homes are without radio or TV these days, but sometimes these facilities do little to encourage children to listen properly. The saying 'Familiarity breeds contempt' may very well apply here. The solution may be to use the *off* button more frequently and when the *on* button is used, to give the programme proper attention. Treat yourself to a break from the chores. Sit down quietly and listen or watch together. Perhaps you can sing or dance to the music, discuss the plot, explain unusual words . . . With your help, the child will be having a true listening experience.

Try making a sound picture. For this you need a cassette recorder and quite a lot of imagination. First think of a situation, then imagine all the noises that combine to make that situation recognisable. Imagine a walk down the High Street. If it is not pedestrianised, there will be the noises of the traffic, perhaps a Police car or an Ambulance in a hurry, footsteps on the pavement, scraps of conversations, maybe a barking dog or even a busker! Of course, all these sounds can be recorded in the street in the real situation. They can also be imitated by various means at home. A 'sound picture' was made in this way by a group of teenagers with learning difficulties. They first went for a walk by the river, and on returning to their classroom, they tried to recreate on tape the sounds they had heard. They used the Slither Box (p. 115) to indicate footsteps on the gravel tow-path. The sound of the wind in the reeds was made by rubbing the palms of their hands together. Someone dabbled his hand in a bowl of water to represent the lapping of the ripples against the bank and, of course, the siren of the tripper boat and the quacking of the ducks could not be left out.

NOISY MOBILES

Dancing Danglement

Quick

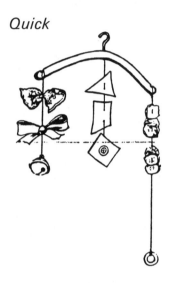

This is a mobile that does not rely on a draught to make it move. It is activated by 'baby power'. When the string is pulled, the mobile will bob about and set all the noisemakers jangling.

A coat-hanger is hung out of reach of the child, but where he can see it easily. An assortment of noisy objects and some colourful ones are tied to the hanger. These might include a bunch of bells, a string of foil milk bottle tops, a rattle, a tassel of brightly-coloured ribbons, cellophane sweet wrappers — tied in the middle to make them look like butterflies . . . Make about three strings of these with one considerably longer than the others. This is the one for the child to pull. Make it easy to hold by tying a ring or cotton reel to the end. Be sure the strings cannot slip off the hanger — either drill holes for them or cut notches in the top. On a plastic hanger, bind the strings in place with Sellotape.

A Bamboo Mobile

Long-lasting

This mobile can be used in two ways: in version 1, the mobile is hung out of reach (like the Dancing Danglement above), and the child pulls a string to make the sound; in version 2, as shown, it is hung within reach for a 'hands on' experience. In this case the child can run his hands along the line of bamboo tubes to make them strike together. This mobile is weather resistant, so is suitable for hanging outside — on a verandah perhaps, or in the winter from the branches of a bare tree, where it could provide a welcome spot of colour in a dreary winter landscape.

Materials
- A length of broomstick or thick dowel for support.
- Bamboo garden canes . . . say two.

- An old knitting needle.
- Paint. Acrylic is best, but poster will do.
- Polyurethane varnish.
- Thin nylon cord for suspending the support.
- Strong, thin thread for hanging the bamboo sections.
- Beads — optional, but they make the bamboo sections hang better and look pretty.
- Tools — a small saw, two drills, a craft knife, sandpaper.

Method

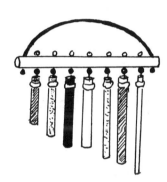

Divide the bamboo canes into separate sections by cutting about 10 mm ($\frac{1}{4}''$) above each joint. The sections will be different lengths and thicknesses. Discard any split or faulty ones and keep about eight to ten of the best. With a craft knife, scratch away all the waxy surface on the outside of each section. (Work away from yourself, and take care.) It is important to remove all the waxy surface or the paint will not stick properly, and will chip off when the sections knock together. Rub each section with sandpaper to ensure that the surface is smooth and clean. Drill a small hole, just large enough to take the hanging thread, down through the joint at the top of each section. Remove the pith in the middle with a knitting needle. Hold the cane up to your eye and you should now be able to see right through it. Poke the hanging thread through the hole in the top of the section and out through the bottom. Tie a very large knot on the end, or better still, thread it through a small bead to prevent it from pulling out through the hole in the joint. Paint all the bamboo sections in bright colours and, when they are dry, protect each with at least two coats of polyurethane varnish. Decide how you would like them to hang and arrange them in a row. Leave a gap between each — about the width of a section — and measure the space they occupy. Cut the broomstick (or dowel) hanger about 8 cm (3″) longer. Drill holes at appropriate intervals along it, one for each section of bamboo and one each end for the suspending cord. Tie each section to the hanger. If you use beads, thread one as a spacer between a section and the hanger, and

111

perhaps one on the top (as in the illustration) to make sure the section will not drop off. Finally, attach the suspending cord and a pull string if you are making version 1.

A Circular Mobile a Child Can Sit Inside

Quick

Like the two mobiles above, this one also rewards a child for making an effort! In this case, he sits surrounded by potential noisemakers which seem to invite him to give them a biff.

The hanger for this mobile is a large plastic hoop. It must be suspended horizontally from three or four points, and hung at the correct height to encircle the child's head like a giant halo. Noisemakers dangle from the hoop. Here are three suggestions.

- Use balloons. To keep the child guessing, put a few grains of rice inside some, but not all. The rice will make a soft rustling sound. Keep the strings fairly short or they will tangle.
- Copy the mobile made by a teacher at Linden Bennet School. Cardboard rolls (from baking foil or paper towels) were painted in bright colours or covered with foil paper. A bell was hung inside some of them.
- At White Lodge Centre, Margaret Gillman bedizened her hoop with tin lids. (No sharp edges!) The spacing was important. Hitting one lid should make it swing against its neighbours.

HOMEMADE NOISEMAKERS

Here are some noisemakers that can be made from odds and ends. Their size and noisiness can easily be adapted, so there should be something suitable for every child, however special their need. Some of the noisemakers can be shaken with one hand, others encourage the use of two. Most can be manipulated by children who have restricted movements.

Making a noise is one of the universal pleasures of childhood. Being able to shake, rattle or bang on a drum can give more than just sensory pleasure. To be in control of the sound he makes can give a child a little more confidence in himself, and a lovely sense of power — especially if the sounds he makes produce a reaction in others. Think of the horrible noise of a knife scraping across a plate, and the way it sets our teeth on edge! The noisemakers suggested here are much more socially acceptable. Used purposefully, as in a band, or being played in time to the radio, these simple 'instruments' can help children to listen more carefully, and may even help to improve their co-ordination and powers of concentration.

A Rattle from a Fruit Juice Bottle

Instant

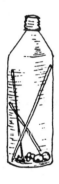

This rattle is ideal for a child who has just learnt to sit up, or for an older, gentle child. Its size, light weight and transparency give it child appeal. Its owner is likely to spend ages shaking the bottle, watching the contents bob about inside, and trying to make the loudest possible noise.

Wash the bottle thoroughly, and make sure it is really dry. If any moisture remains, it will form condensation, and the contents may stick together and not rattle properly. Practically any filling may be used but, in the interests of safety, it is best to stick to edible items like spaghetti, rice, lentils, etc. If you are certain the child will not manage to undo the lid, a few brightly-coloured buttons and some scraps of foil paper will look more attractive, and possibly make a louder noise. Once the contents are inside, the lid must be fixed on securely with polystyrene cement (e.g. U-Hu). Make sure this is set before offering the rattle to the child.

A Strong Rattle from a Washing-up Liquid Bottle

Instant, or Quick (if painted)

This is much more robust than the one above, and will stand a heavier filling. For safety reasons, fix the stopper in place with polystyrene cement, and cut off the small plastic lid and the loop which attaches it to the bottle. The bottle will now have a hole in the top. This will add to its attraction, for it can also be used as a puffer.

The outside of the bottle can be made more decorative by scrubbing off the printing with wire wool, then decorating it with a pattern painted with

Humbrol enamel. This paint is quite safe for children, dries quickly, does an excellent cover-up job, and will not crack when the bottle is squeezed.

A Loud Rattle from an Inverted Treacle Tin

Quick

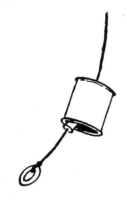

This rattle resembles a crude ship's bell. Its special feature is that it is capable of generating plenty of decibels! It can be either hand held, or tied to a suitable point such as a cot play bar or, for a child lying on the floor, the rung of a chair. When tied to something, it can make a useful rattle for children who tend to throw or drop their toys. I used the prototype, hand held, when I wanted to attract the attention of a group of children, and signal a change of activity.

Remove the lid from the tin and save it. It has a nicely turned lip — no sharp edges — and could come in handy for another toy! (e.g. the Sit Inside Mobile, p. 112). Wash the tin thoroughly and dry it. Punch a hole in the centre of the bottom. Push from the outside inwards so that the rough edges are inside. Thread about 45 cm (18″) of string or piping cord through the hole. The latter is better — it looks more attractive and is soft to feel. Leave a tail of cord (for the clapper), then tie a large knot in the cord to prevent it from pulling out of the tin, and another knot outside — to keep the cord in place and stop it from disappearing inside. Make the clapper by threading a *large* wooden bead, or a cotton reel or a wooden brick with a hole drilled in it, onto the tail of cord. Tie a knot to prevent it from falling off. Make sure the clapper is in the right position to strike the tin, and produce the maximum noise. Tie a ring to the end of the tail to make it easier to grasp. Possibly, decorate the tin with Humbrol enamel.

A Jumbo Shaker

Quick

Rosemary Hemmett,
Toy Librarian

Do you ever search in vain for a really large rattle? This one can be used by an older child for whom 'baby' rattles are too small and fragile.

Rosemary uses a tough plastic salad shaker that looks like two colanders joined together by a hinge. Normally, freshly washed lettuce is placed inside and rapidly shaken to remove all the surplus water. Replace the lettuce with ping-pong balls or, better still, cat balls (each with a bell inside) from the pet shop. Tie the two halves of the salad shaker together. Bind round the handles and tie at intervals round the edge. You now have a large, strong rattle that can be carried about or hung up to be biffed or kicked.

Special Rattles for 'Frail' Children

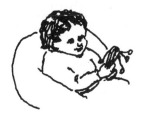

Tic-tac box. The need here is for extra small and light rattles. One teacher uses a Tic-Tac sweet container, puts in a few grains of rice and seals down the lid by binding the container with plastic tape.

A small dumbbell-shaped rattle can be made by using part of the tube of a felt pen. Cut it to the length required. A strong thread, or round elastic, is passed down the centre and a bell tied to each end. If necessary, the rattle can be encased in fabric.

An empty film carton can soon be transformed into a small cylindrical rattle. A parent who attends the toy library showed me one she had made for her little daughter. She put a bell inside the carton, replaced the lid, and covered the whole thing with a crochet cover worked in fine, brightly-coloured wools. The cover made the rattle visually attractive, less slippery to hold, and made certain the lid could not come off.

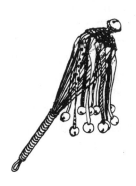

An unusual twirly rattle — highly acclaimed by all the children to when I have given one — has been invented by Alison Wisbeach. Its skeleton is a small metal egg whisk. Short lengths of brightly-coloured ribbon, each with a bell stitched to one end, are sewn to each loop of wire. When the whisk is twirled, these fly out like the chairs in a fairground chair-a-plane. To ensure that this happens, the ribbons must be prevented from crowding together at the top of the whisk. This can be done by backstitching in wool over each loop of wire in turn, so forming a web to block in the end of the whisk. Press the strands together, and keep them in place with a few stitches between the loops of wire.

A Slither Box

Quick

This rattle makes an unusual sound. It is used in the sound picture described on p. 109 to imitate the noise of footsteps on gravel. Tilted more slowly, it can make

115

you think of waves breaking on a stony beach. It contains fish grit (used in aquaria), and the feeling of the weight being transferred from one hand to the other is intriguing to children. When one boy first held it, he spent ages slowly turning it over and over in an attempt to make a continuous sound. Its unusual shape and sound makes it attractive to older children who have thoroughly explored the possibilities of other percussion instruments. Be generous with the papier mâché layers that cover it, and it will be very strong.

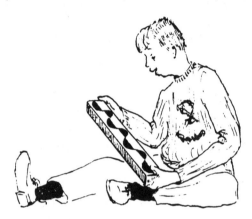

Use a fairly large *flat* cardboard box — the longer the better. Put in a few spoonfuls of fish grit or, for the softer sound, use rice, dried peas, etc. — experiment! Next, thoroughly cover the box with many layers of strips of torn newspaper and PVA adhesive, watered down for economy! Wait for the box to be thoroughly dry. Cover the newsprint with a coat of pale emulsion paint. When that is dry, decorate the box with a bold pattern using Humbrol enamel, or water-based paint, and add a final protective cover of polyurethane varnish.

Bell Shakers with an Easy-grip Handle

Quick

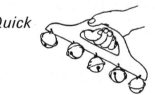

For children who find it difficult to grasp, it can be worthwhile making a pair of bell shakers from wooden workbag handles obtainable from a craft shop or car boot sale! Along the bottom edge of the handles (where the bag is usually attached), drill a few holes far enough apart for the bells to hang independently of each other.

Clappers

Quick

Use two pieces of wood—thick enough to have handles screwed to them and about $15 \times 7\frac{1}{2}$ cm ($6 \times 3''$). Round off the corners and rub thoroughly with sandpaper. Screw a handle to the centre of each. Some children may need a doorknob, others a long cupboard door handle. See what is on offer at the local DIY store, and choose the most suitable for the child in mind.

Scraper

Instant or Quick

In its instant form, the perfect scraper is an old-fashioned washboard. Now and then one of these can still be found in junk shops, and very occasionally at car boot or jumble sales. Show a child how to rub a drum stick across the ridges to make an unusual and interesting sound. Better still, dispense with the stick, and put thimbles on his fingers. This way he will have a close affinity with the sound he is making, and will experience a delicious tingling sensation in his fingertips.

If you like the washboard idea, but have searched the junk shops in vain, try making one from some ridged material. A trip to the DIY store could produce fluted pelmet board, ridged doorstep protector or some other unlikely material for a toy! Beware of sharp edges which, of course, must be covered. One parent mounted some metal with narrow corrugations on wood and surrounded the edges with beading, like a picture frame. The result was a heavy, but very strong and safe percussion instrument.

For Children with Poor Hand Control

It is possible that none of the ideas above can be comfortably manipulated by a child with very poor hand function. One of the simple suggestions below, contributed by Christine Cousins and John Gould, might help.

Make bell bracelets. Use a sweat band or a strip of stretchy material with Velcro attached to each end. Sew bells (from a pet shop) all round it. Put it on the most controllable part of the child's body—wrist, ankle, forehead?

117

Suspend a tambourine within easy biffing range. Make sure that it is secured at three points, so that it will not swing or twist.

Make sand blocks for a child who can only use one hand. Fix a sheet of sandpaper to the table with masking tape. Cover a wooden brick with sandpaper for the child to rub on the sheet with his able hand.

A Trail of Noisy Objects

Instant

Pam Courtney, Teacher

When children are constantly on the move, they are exercising both their muscles and their brains. As they explore their surroundings, they learn from all the new experiences and discoveries that come their way. A child with a visual handicap may need to be coaxed from the security of her own special corner, and the same reluctance to explore can also be a problem with those slow learners who seem perfectly happy to stay put. Without help, such children are unlikely to develop either physically or mentally as quickly as they should.

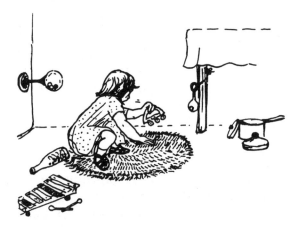

One way of increasing such a child's self-confidence, and persuading her to 'have a go', might be to follow Pam's suggestion and lay a trail of noisy objects. Her intention is to lure the child from one noisemaker to the next, using anything that has child-appeal. The trail could include favourite sound-producing toys and rattles, the ever-popular saucepan and wooden spoon, or even an unfamiliar junk rattle like a few stones in a tin. At first the child needs to be introduced to the idea of moving from one noisemaker to the next. Perhaps she starts by playing happily with a familiar rattle. When this begins to pall, her attention may be attracted by someone starting to play a xylophone softly, fairly close to her, but just out of reach. If she wants to know more about this fascinating new sound, she must move towards it (perhaps coaxed by some encouraging words). At a later stage, when she feels more confident, the trail of noisy objects can be laid in a line across the floor, or round the edge of the carpet, for her to discover in her own time. If the child is visually handicapped, this activity will give her an idea of the layout of the room, and help her to find her way around.

TOYS WITH AN INBUILT NOISE

Octopully

Long-lasting

A short entry in an early edition of Information Exchange described how an enterprising teacher in a Special Care Unit filled old tights with crunched-up newspaper and draped them over the children. What a splendid 'instant' idea — surely it could be developed into an attractive long-lasting toy!

The multi-armed octopus seemed the ideal model for such a toy, and soon the usual hotch potch of materials was transformed into the Octopully. Unlike the real thing, this version has tentacles that are intended to be explored by inquisitive fingers, and on the end of each is a bag containing a rattle, squeaker, bell, etc. It has been given the 'thumbs up' by children with multiple disabilities, who have obligingly tested it for me.

The Octopully can be hung up (possibly on elastic to make it more challenging to grab), tied to the side of a cot, draped across a play table, or just left lying about on the floor to be discovered by a child who, in all probability, will feel motivated to roll, 'swim' or crawl towards it.

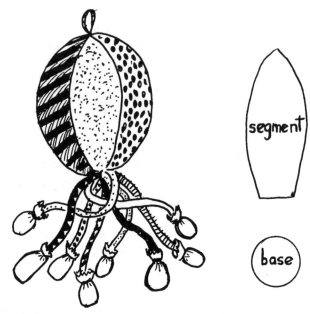

Materials

- Scraps of material for the body and for the bags at the end of the tentacles.
- Short length of piping or nylon cord for the hanging loop.
- Polyester filling.
- Small circle of card for the base of the body.
- Lengths of material for the tentacles could be:
    wide, strong ribbon, flat or plaited;
    thick wool, plaited;
    bubbly plastic, cut in strips about 5 cm (2″) wide and plaited;
    a string of large beads loosely threaded on nylon cord;
    pyjama cord or wool braid, decorated with buttons firmly sewn on;
    stitched tubes of material with a pleasant feel and/or bright colour. (Seam together the long edges of a strip of material, right side inside. Attach a safety pin to one end, poke it in the tube, and gradually work it along until it comes out at the other end, turning the tube the right side out in the process);
- A selection of noisemakers in containers for the tentacle ends, *see* fillings suggested for 'Rattles in Pairs' on p. 128.

Method

Refer to the diagram and make a paper pattern. A suitable size for the body of the Octopully is about 20 cm (8″) long. Using strong, brightly-coloured material, cut out six body segments. Stitch them together, stopping just short of the top. By doing this, you will have left a small hole for the insertion of the hanging loop. Push the ends of the loop into the hole and knot them together inside the body. By hand, neaten the top of the Octopully. Turn in any raw edges and sew round it several times. This will also make sure that the loop will never pull out.

Make eight tentacles (suggested size 30 cm or 12″) and sew them to the open end of the Octopully.

Cut out the circular base in card, and cover it with a larger circle of material. Keep the material in position with a few criss-crossing threads (which will be hidden inside the body once the base is attachod).

Now stuff the Octopully with polyester fibre, then close the hole with the circular base, keeping it in place with at least two rounds of ladder stitch.

Make eight bags for the ends of the tentacles. Fill them with noisemakers of your choice and stitch one (firmly!) to the end of each tentacle.

Friendly Rattlesnakes

These peculiar reptiles resemble real ones in overall shape but, unlike them, they have noisemakers distributed throughout their long bodies. They can be made very quickly as a temporary toy — soon out-grown — or, stitched with care, they can become a child's treasured possession.

A Quick Version

Marianne Willemsen van Witsen,
Toymaker,
Holland

Marianne collects several cardboard tubes. She puts rice inside them to make the rattle. She blocks off the ends of the tubes with circles of paper, like jam pot covers, and glues them in place. For a slightly stronger and more decorative snake, the tubes can be covered with fabric. They are inserted, one by one, into the leg of a pair of tights. A tie of ribbon or thick wool separates each section, so that the snake will bend. It is surprising how many tubes the leg will hold if it is stretched tightly over each one.

121

PLAY HELPS

Quick

John Fisher, author
of 'Toys to Grow With'

A Sock Snake

The skin of this rattle snake is just a long sock. For its 'innards' John suggests:

- some crackly material, like a potato crisp bag, a foil bag from a packet of tea or coffee, or even a deflated helium balloon;
- a rattle or two;
- a squeaky toy;
- something soft — like the other sock rolled up.

Method

First choose a soft item, and stuff it into the toe of the sock. Tie it in place with strong thread and a double knot, and trim off the ends. In goes the next item, again firmly tied in place . . . and so on until the sock is filled, ending with another soft item. In the hands of a baby, this toy will be waved about, and he will probably hit himself with it. For this reason, it is wise to put the soft, squashy items at both ends and keep the hard rattles for the middle.

Long-lasting

The Rattlesnake as a More Robust Toy

A few years ago I was asked to make some toys for some overseas children I had never met. I knew they had learning difficulties and were all under five; also that there might be times during the day when their play would be unsupervised. Therefore, a toy that was as strong and safe as possible was required. After various experiments, I came up with an impressively long snake that was both noisy and tactile.

At the time my 'grot box' contained some tough plastic pill bottles with safety caps. Putting a few dried peas in one of these gave it an instant rattle with a splendid clatter. The skin of the snake was made from pieces of strong material joined together patchwork fashion. I began to experiment, and found that a snake which had eaten an exclusive diet of pill bottles was too noisy. Of course, this could be a good point for a child with a hearing loss, but I was considering the nerves of the adults! This is why the 'feely' sections were introduced. I soon had a production line going, and a box full of friendly snakes. Someone visiting the children reported that, after about three months' heavy use, they were grubby, but still intact.

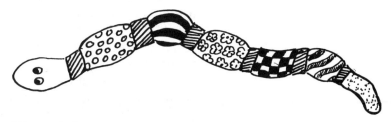

Materials

- Small pieces of very strong, colourful fabric for the skin.
- A little polyester fibre for the head and the tail.
- A collection of tactile objects. Select suitable ones from the list on p. 149.
- Some rattles, and other noisemakers. Suggestions for fillings on p. 129.

Method

Make the snake about a metre long. This gives plenty of scope for interesting 'innards'. Lay out the contents of the snake in the order in which you will use them, grading them in size. Alternate a tactile section with a noisy one. Arrange the different pieces of fabric in an attractive way, possibly putting a narrow strip of the same colour between each. I found this gave the snake a pleasing appearance, and acted as a hinge between the sections, making the toy suitably floppy. When the time came to fill the snake I left these strips empty.

Next, cut each section of fabric the right size to fit the article it will later contain — large things near the head, graduating down towards the tail. Each section of fabric must be wide enough to wrap round a hard, unyielding rattle, with a bit extra for the seam allowance. The length of each piece will vary.

Rattles should fit fairly snugly inside their section, but tactile objects should have room to move around, as in a feely bag. Don't forget the seam allowance at each end, where one section joins to the next. Join all the pieces of fabric together in a long strip. Fold

123

this in half, right sides together, and pin at all the places where the fabrics join. Round off the head and the tail of the snake. Stitch along the side seam and round the end of the tail. Turn the snake skin right side out. Stuff the tail with polyester fibre. Stitch across the snake skin to keep it in place. (If you have used narrow strips of unifying fabric between the sections, as in the illustration, stitch across again just before the next section.) Continue like this, adding the contents as you go. Finally, stuff the head with polyester fibre, close the seam with ladder stitch, and add felt features to give the snake a benign expression.

A Chain in a Bottle

Almost instant

Hettie Whitby,
Teacher of Visually
Impaired Children

This is a simple but intriguing toy — one of the best I have come across. If you are familiar with Winnie-the-Pooh and his friends, you will know the story of Eeyore's birthday present. Pooh and Piglet meant to give him a jar of honey and a balloon, but one got accidentally popped and the other absentmindedly eaten. He ended up with a damp bit of rubbery rag and an empty honey jar. To his infinite satisfaction, Eeyore found that he could put the popped balloon in the honey jar, *and* take it out again! His friends left him happily repeating this action over and over again. This toy has the same appeal — now you see it, now you don't!

The bottle is a discarded plastic one that has a handle moulded into it. In its working life, it probably contained fabric softener. It is a pretty blue and, of course, the handle makes it easy to grasp. The chain can be bought from the local ironmongers (or DIY store). The length needed is about twice the height of the bottle. In theory, the chain should stick to the bottom of the bottle with a blob of Araldite. I must confess mine did not. Perhaps the bottle was damp! It was a simple matter to stitch the chain to the bottom of the bottle by squinting through the neck and poking a long needle, threaded with button thread, in through one side of the bottle, through the end link and out through the other side. I repeated the process several times, in effect binding the chain to the bottom of the bottle. A child can have fun dropping the chain in the bottle and shaking it out again, but for most children it is better to go one step further and tie a ring or a cotton reel to the other end of the chain. This makes it easy to hold and prevents it from totally disappearing inside the bottle. Offer this peculiar toy to a child who has just learnt to sit independently, or to an older one who has a craze on 'doodle' toys, and you are sure to have a happy and satisfied customer!

A See-Saw Marble Run

Long-lasting

This is a 'general purpose' toy. It appeals to eyes, ears and hands. Children of many ages will spend a considerable time tipping the see-saw from one side to the other for the pleasure of watching—and listening to—the marbles as they scuttle down the central track. As with all see-saws, it works with a

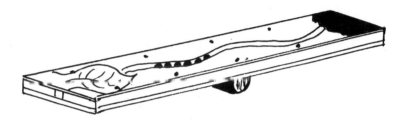

simple balancing action. The track, covered with perspex, curves in a gentle wavy line and the marbles travel from one end to the other, their speed varying according to the tilt of the see-saw. Once children understand the principle, they like to tip the see-saw very gradually to make the marbles travel at a snail's pace. (Make them go too slowly, and some will separate from the pack and roll back to base.)

Michael Wason adapted this toy to represent a creepy crawly caterpillar. One end of the perspex was painted brown—to represent the earth—and on the other was painted a leaf. The marbles could shelter under the 'earth', then scuttle down the track to eat the 'leaf', and back again, ad infinitum.

Note
Perspex is expensive. For a cheaper version for an individual child of known habits, try using thick industrial polythene, or, *if safe*, dispense with the cover altogether. Just issue the marbles at play time and collect them all up afterwards.

Materials
- About ten marbles. Small ones will do.
- One strip of plywood, about $\frac{3}{4}$ metre long, and thicker than the diameter of the marbles.
- Another strip of plywood, the same length, but slightly wider. It is for the base, so can be thinner.
- A block of wood, for the centre balancing point of the see-saw — say $7\frac{1}{2}$ cm (3″) × 10–12 cm (4–4$\frac{3}{4}$″).
- A strip of perspex, the same size as the plywood base, to cover the top, and keep the marbles in place.
- Some screws, paint, masking tape, wood glue.

Method
Cut the thick ply into two pieces with a gentle wavy line down the middle — a band saw does this job well. Do not make the curves too pronounced or the marbles will not run smoothly. With masking tape, temporarily fix one half of the see-saw track to the ply base. Leave a narrow gap, just wide enough to take the marbles comfortably, then tape the other half of the see-saw track to the base. When you are quite sure the marbles are running up and down the track with the maximum efficiency, mark the positions of the two halves of the see-saw track, but don't glue them down just yet. Next, round off the base of the balancing block. Temporarily fix the block to the centre of the base (double sided Sellotape?) and try out the tilt of the see-saw. If this is too steep, the marbles will rush too quickly from one end to the other, and the block will need to be made a little lower. When you are satisfied all is well, glue the block to the base. Countersink, say, four screws through the base and into the block for extra strength. Sandpaper the sides of the track and the top of the base where the marbles will roll. Temporarily fix the two halves of the track to their lines on the base. Test again that the marbles will run freely. If so, screw and glue the sides to the base. Make small plugs of plywood for each end of the track to prevent the marbles from escaping. Sandpaper all the surfaces and paint them. When the paint is thoroughly dry, insert the marbles and cover the top with perspex. Fix it in place with plenty of screws.

Noisy Busy Board

Long-lasting

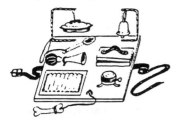

This is a toy with plenty of scope for ingenuity. Basically, it is just a sheet of sturdy ply, whatever shape and size you choose, with an assortment of noise-makers screwed to it. Some, like the motor horn and the bicycle bell in the illustration, might need a firm touch to set them going; others, like the bell and the bone scraper, can give a noisy reward for less physical effort. The number of items on the board, their spacing, simplicity and noisiness can all be governed by the needs of the child in question. A wander round the pet shop, DIY store or local ironmongers is sure to produce plenty of attractive noisemakers suitable for mounting. For anyone with an electrical bent, a battery-driven bell or a morse buzzer could be included.

See also
  Fiddle Toys, p. 144
  Amorphous Beanbag, p. 148
  Manx Feely Cushion, p. 148

LISTENING GAMES

Plink Plonk

Instant

We all know why mothers attach toys with lengths of ribbon to the sides of cots and prams. The baby who is active and curious is for ever throwing his toys on the floor for someone else to retrieve. Even if Mum is cross, at least the baby knows he is holding her attention! Some children with special needs could miss out on this traditional activity. The game of Plink Plonk can be a simple way of helping them to share the experience.

The game is nothing more than giving a child the chance to drop all kinds of objects into (or onto) something so that an interesting noise will be made. As a bonus, it gives plenty of practice in grasping and releasing, and is an ideal way of presenting the child with an assortment of objects to feel. These can be heavy or light, hard or soft, and have differing textural feels. A collection of any odd objects will do for the game — cotton reels, conkers, fir cones, clothes pegs, hair curlers, smooth stones . . . the list can go on and on. Containers to drop them into might be a large cardboard box (difficult to miss!) for a dull thud, a biscuit tin for a clank, a bucket, plastic or galvanised, or even the kitchen sink.

The game can be made a little more difficult for an older child by giving him a tube for the items to slide down. This version encourages the use of both hands, one to post the objects and the other to direct the tube in the right direction. It is sometimes possible to find very long tubes in soft furnishing departments of large stores. These are thrown away once the material they held has been sold. They are the ultimate for this game, and can encourage some careful listening. The length of the tube causes a time lag between posting the object and the satisfying clonk as it reaches its destination.

Echoes

Instant

This can be a good game to play at odd moments, on car journeys etc. It consists of imitating a familiar sound like a clock ticking, a fire engine, a car horn or an animal noise. You make the sound and your child echoes it. Then perhaps he makes the sound for you to copy. Making a noise to produce a real echo, (in a valley, or walking through a tunnel?) can prompt a child to listen really intently.

The Robot Game

Instant

The child pretends to be a robot, moving stiffly around the room. He is controlled by a code of agreed sounds. Perhaps, when you clap your hands twice he takes two steps forward. Stamp your foot once and he must take a step backwards. A bell might indicate a forward movement, and a drum for reverse. Keep the instruments out of sight, so that the child must really listen for his instructions. If the game goes well, you might increase the number of noises — shake a rattle for a right turn, snap your fingers for 'sit down'!

Rattles in Pairs to make a Sound Matching Game

Quick

Collect an even number of containers with lids — at least six. Film cartons, little plastic pots (used to hold potato salad etc.) or even a collection of Nesquick tins, as used by the nursery children at White Lodge Centre, might do. Whatever you use, it is essential that the containers are identical, and that the contents will be invisible. Arrange the containers in pairs, and put a small quantity of the same noisemaker in each pair. Replace the lids and glue or tape them on. The containers are muddled up. The children take it in turns to choose two, shake them, and hope that they will match in sound. If they do not, the containers are returned to the table, and someone else tries his luck. An observant child who has been listening hard will notice which sound each container has made and, when his turn comes, will probably be able to pick a pair.

Suitable fillings for the containers might be rice, dried peas, butter beans, pebbles, coins, bells, buttons, sand, or milkbottle tops. It is important that the pairs of sounds are distinguishable from each other. Rice and lentils, shaken in the same kind of container can sound identical. Consider the safety factor very carefully when using items from this list. You know best the habits of the children who will use your game, and if they are likely to remove the lids and make a meal of the contents.

This sound matching game can be interesting for any age from toddler to teenager. At the younger end, make the sounds very distinctive and not too numerous. Use, for example, sand, bells and dried peas. At the older end, use more pairs of sounds and make them less easily distinguishable. Some teenagers are likely to be curious about the contents of the containers, and with their stronger hands may easily remove the lids. This was certainly the case with one group. No known glue could defeat them! The problem was solved by covering the containers, in this case film cartons, with strips of newspaper and paste. When dry, they were all painted the same colour. The children could no longer *see* the lids, so the urge to take them off disappeared.

Start-stop games

Instant

These well-loved games are popular with all children at a certain stage in their lives. They encourage children to listen to the music (live or canned), and react appropriately when it stops. If necessary, the rules can be adjusted a little and the pace reduced so that all can join in the fun.

Musical Chairs

Have a chair for each child. Arrange these either in a circle with a space between each, or in a line with alternate chairs facing in opposite directions. Before the game begins, remove a chair so that one child must stand up. When the music starts, the children walk round the chairs. When it suddenly stops, they must all try to sit down. The child now left standing is 'out'. Another chair is removed, and the game continues until two children are competing for one chair. When the music stops, the child who sits on it is the winner.

Alternative Version where No-one is 'Out'

This version is hilarious, but can become quite rough. The chairs are removed as usual, but when the music stops *everyone* must sit down. This means using the knees of those fortunate enough to find an empty chair. Towards the end of the game, sitters are not so lucky, because everyone is piled up on their knees!

Musical Hats

First make a collection of hats, the more outlandish the better. The children stand in a circle, facing the back of the child in front. All but one must wear a hat. When the music plays all walk forward and the hatless child grabs a hat from the head in front. This sets off a chain reaction as each hatless child in turn tries to cover his head. When the music stops, the then hatless child is out. Another hat is removed from the circle (there must always be one short), and so the game continues. This is a popular game with older children (even with adults!), for they enjoy wearing the ridiculous hats and, when they are 'out', it is even better because they can laugh at everyone else. This can be quite a rough game as it nears its climax, so watch out!

Musical Mats

While the music plays, the children run round in a circle, at one place jumping over a mat. When the music stops the last one over the mat is 'out'.

Musical Statues

This is yet another version of the musical start-stop game. The children dance around and, when the music stops, they must instantly become a statue, and keep absolutely still until the music starts again. This calls for considerable balancing skill. You can either withdraw the first child that wobbles, or play uncompetitively and praise the best statue. To praise is kinder and usually leads to more imaginative efforts and greater fun.

Command games

Like the games above, these also call for attentive listening. Some may be new to you.

Traffic Lights

This game is best played in a large room and with several children. If the leader calls out 'Red', the children must sit down, for 'Amber' they must stand still, and for 'Green' they must run about.

Do This, Do That

This is a less lively game than Traffic Lights. It can be adapted to suit many situations and can even be played by children in bed. It certainly encourages attentive listening. The leader says 'Do this' and performs a simple action, such as clapping her hands or pointing to the ceiling. On this command, all the children copy her. If she says 'Do that' they must ignore her new action and continue to do the previous one.

Simon Says

This game is similar to the one above, and makes a useful alternative. If an instruction from the leader is preceded by 'Simon says . . .' it must be obeyed. Without these two magic words, all instructions must be ignored, e.g. 'Simon says clap your hands'. Everyone starts clapping. The next instruction might be 'Point to the door'. The children must continue to clap their hands, because Simon did not tell them to do otherwise.

Other group games

Animal Treasure Hunt

This is a very noisy game and best played in a big room with a large group of children. They are divided into teams, each representing an animal with a noisy call—cat, dog, cow, lion, etc. They stand facing a wall and hide their eyes while butter-beans are hidden all round the room. The children search for the beans. When they find one they may not touch it, but must make their animal call to attract the attention of the team leader, who is the only one allowed to collect it. When this has been done, the child runs off to search for another bean. The winning team, of course, is the one with the most beans. To make the game more difficult, use rice or dried peas.

How Warm You Are

One child goes out of the room. The rest decide on an article he is to touch when he comes back . . . e.g. a cushion (easy) or a particular flower in a vase (difficult). When the child enters the room, everyone starts to sing 'How warm you are' (over and over again) to the tune of Auld Lang Syne. When the child is near the object, the singing must be loud; if he moves away, the children must sing softly. ('Warm' might change to 'cold'.)

He is finally guided to the object by the loudness of the singing, and the game continues with another child going out of the room . . .

The Ring Master

One child is blindfolded and stands in the centre of a circle of children. They dance round him until he cries 'Stop!' He points to someone in the circle and says 'Make the noise of a lion' (horse, cat, mouse, dog, etc.). He must try to guess which child is making the noise.

The Bell Game

This game has obvious hazards, and must be well supervised and played in a large, unobstructed space. It can be great fun for older, energetic children. All the children but one are blindfolded and given a whacker made out of rolled-up newspaper. The odd child has bells hung round his waist, ankles, wrists . . . wherever convenient. He must dodge between the whackers and try to get from one end of the play area to the other.

QUIETER LISTENING GAMES

Giant's Treasure

The giant sits in the middle of the room, guarding his treasure. (A little bell or other noisemaker.) He is blindfolded. The children sit in a large circle round him. The leader signals to one child, who must try to creep forward very stealthily and try to steal the giant's treasure. If the giant hears him coming, he must point in the direction of the sound. If he points correctly, the thieving child must return to his place, and the leader chooses someone else to have a try.

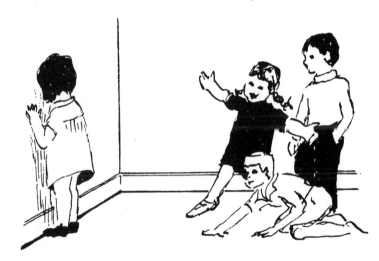

Grandmother's Footsteps

One child is grandmother and stands at one end of the room, facing the wall. The rest of the children stand with their backs to the opposite wall. When given the signal, they must creep forward and try to touch Grandmother. If she hears a sound, she can turn round. If she *sees* a child move, she can send him back to the start. This game needs firm refereeing or heated arguments can arise! It is always a favourite though, and calls for concentration and balance from the children and acute listening from Grandmother. It is best played in a large room.

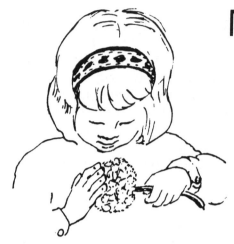

Making the most of TOUCH

THE PURPOSE OF THIS CHAPTER IS TO SUGGEST ways in which all children can be encouraged to use their sense of touch to give them information and fun. The toys and activities below will introduce children to new textures and 'feely' experiences, and may help to make hands more controlled and skilful.

THE IMPORTANCE OF LEARNING TO TOUCH

For visually handicapped children the senses of hearing and touch must obviously be developed as fully as possible to compensate for their impaired sight. The more the use of these senses can be encouraged, the quicker the child can become less dependent and lead a fuller life. The three-year-old with nimble fingers can sort her socks into pairs by feeling the patterns on the legs, and even tights can be put on with less of a battle if she can first sort out the gusset from the heels. Recognising toys by their feel, and realising where she is by touching the textured wallpaper or cold kitchen tiles are skills she will soon learn. As she grows older she will gradually discover how to dress and undress herself, managing buttons, zips, and poppers on the way. She will go shopping and learn to sort and identify coins, and at school she will learn Braille. For this she will need not only a good memory, but also very sensitive fingertips to help her distinguish between the various combinations of the six tiny dots which make up the Braille symbols. Such sensitivity may be helped by using the toys, activities and games that follow.

Now consider a child who finds mobility difficult as his legs are his handicap. If he can be given the opportunity to train his hands to be nimble and creative, he will find many ways of enjoying his leisure time.

Sometimes a slow-learner or a withdrawn child may need a great deal of encouragement even to perform such simple movements as holding and letting go. Perhaps she can be persuaded to use her hands if the reward is sufficiently enticing. Feely toys can sometimes be successful in this situation.

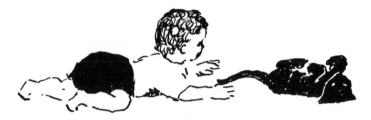

At the other end of the scale is the child who grabs energetically at everything he can reach—sometimes managing to destroy most of it. The homemade toys in this chapter can be made very strong by using double material, extra rows of stitching, etc.

Through our hands we gather information which experience teaches us to interpret. We learn to distinguish between hot and cold, heavy and light, etc. Most important of all, we can use our hands to hold tools. As adults, we often forget the value of these useful members until an accident suddenly makes them useless. Without the help of our fingers we are unable to feed, clothe or clean ourselves, and leisure time can stretch out into a seeming eternity of boredom. With only one hand functioning, it is possible to live a very full life, but with both in working order every desired activity may well be literally within reach.

SOME WAYS OF ENCOURAGING THE SENSE OF TOUCH IN THE HOME

Imagine a baby sitting in his pram. His chief amusement is dropping his toys over the side and watching them fall. Soon his mother becomes fed up with retrieving them and ties them to the side of the pram. Now, in theory, he can pull them up for himself, but it is still the fun of dropping the toy that pleases him — the relaxing of his grasp and the inevitable drop. He has made two wonderful discoveries! He has learnt about the law of gravity, and his own power to make things happen in a comfortingly predictable way.

Another child, however, for whatever reason, may not be able to share in this delightful activity unaided. While he is still physically small, he might be given the chance to grasp and release by being supported over an adult's shoulder. In this position he can drop objects onto a noisy surface like an old tin tray or the stainless steel sink, so that they fall with a satisfying clatter. (An

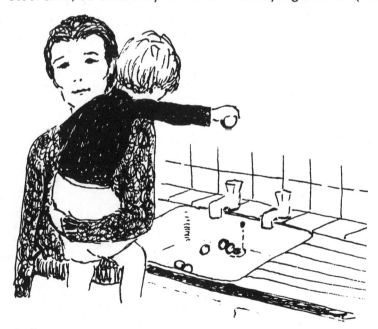

older brother or sister might be persuaded to act as 'salvage man' with the job of reclaiming and returning the dropped toys!) As he is carried around the room, he might be given the opportunity to experience the many different textures on offer — the velvet curtains, the bumpy wallpaper, the cold kitchen tiles, the sun-warmed window ledge . . . and more. These tactile experiences should not happen only once. Think 'textures' and let him touch whatever literally comes to hand as often as possible.

When our pram baby becomes a toddler, he is all agog for more exciting experiences. If he could express himself sufficiently clearly, the average two-year-old would probably vote the garbage pail his favourite toy! Its contents are different every time he gets a chance to investigate it, and even the fact that it is taboo adds to its attraction. One day there might be a cold, shiny empty pickle jar with an interesting smell, curly potato peelings or crackly paper from a box of biscuits. Another day it might hold an egg-box with exciting little pockets in it and a lid to flap about, or bright, smelly orange peel, or brittle egg-shells. Of course, the garbage pail is *not* a toy container, but all the items just mentioned might be given to a child to examine and explore before they end up there. By handling such rubbish under supervision a child can be involved in the daily life of the house. He may never have to peel a potato, but might be given the chance to know that the mash he enjoys for lunch every day does not grow that way.

Unwrapping the Contents of the Shopping Basket

This can be a very useful and informative occupation. Perhaps the shopping can be divided between two

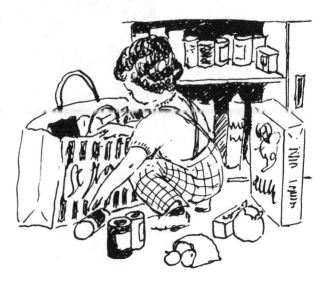

bags, one for fragile items and the other for packets and tins, which are safe for a toddler to handle. Through picking up the various items, he will learn a lot about size, weight, shape and possibly smell. He will have the fun of taking things out of bags, and can learn to recognise the contents by looking at the packaging. He may even be able to pick out special letters like his own initial. During all this inspection his hands will have been turning the articles around, helping him to gain confidence in handling, but not dropping, them.

Hiding Things in Containers

An old handbag can make a perfect toy! Just fill it with a glorious conglomeration of feely articles. (Large buttons; shiny, round conkers; an empty crisp packet; a squeaky toy; an odd sock with a bell tied in it — to name but a few.)

Some children like to wiggle their fingers in a bowl of sand, sawdust, rice, etc, to find a small hidden toy. Others like to fish in a bowl of soapsuds to find a surprise. This can be a good activity for bathtime. Put some bubblebath in a small basin. All the inevitable drips and splashes then fall harmlessly into the big bath where they can be put to their proper use!

FOCUSING ON HANDS

Hands! What incredible appendages they are! Like our miraculous eyes and ears, we take them for granted. Consider the average day. Between getting up and going to bed, our hands will have helped us with washing, dressing, eating, turning knobs, holding things, writing — pen in hand or with modern technology, reading Braille . . . this list of uses could fill this page. Hands are also a vital part of our body language. Through them we can reinforce the meaning of our words. Even one finger can be used to point to something for a child to fetch us, or it can be used in an admonishing manner — 'Don't you *dare* do that again'! Our fingers might be compared to tentacles

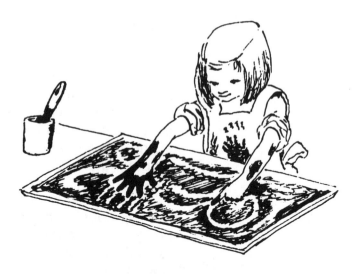

or feelers. We use them to grasp, pull, poke, twist, pick up tiny things and to hold and manipulate tools. No wonder we spend so much time helping the children in our care to make the best use of their hands.

Hand Prints

Quick

People who work and play with brain-damaged children are often looking for new ways of encouraging them to focus on different parts of their bodies, and so help them to understand which bit does what! Making a hand (or foot) print is one way of concentrating a child's attention on that part of him. Hands can be smeared with a fairly thick mixture of powder paint and then used to print their shape on a piece of paper. Alternatively, each hand can be placed flat on the paper while you draw round it. The child can take his time, flattening out his hand and spreading his fingers. Then comes the best bit when he experiences a delightful tingling sensation as your pencil traces round his fingers. Try it!

Hand prints are often cut out and used for classroom decoration. At Linden Bennet School each child in the class makes several pairs of hand prints and a pair of foot prints. These are cut out and arranged on large sheets of paper as giant flowers. The foot prints,

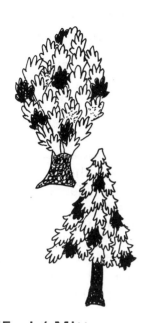

together with a photograph of the child go in the centre of the flower and the hand prints are arranged all around to make the petals.

At Dysart School the body of a large bird is drawn on sugar paper and the outline filled in with overlapping hand-prints, pointing towards the tail, to represent feathers.

At other schools cut-out hand prints are used to make very effective trees. In Autumn they are made in red, yellow and brown to represent the seasonal colours. The hand prints are mounted on paper in the shape of a tree with the fingers pointing upwards. In December there is a call for more hand prints, dark green this time. They can be mounted, fingers pointing downwards, to represent a Christmas tree.

'Feely' Mitts

Quick

(Especially suitable for children with severe visual impairment.) Sorting mitt shapes into pairs can be a useful introduction to other tactile games. The shapes are large, so there is plenty of surface to feel. The pairing process is not as easy as you might think, especially for children who are not yet acquainted with a range of textile textures. If there are many pairs of mitts, the sorting out can be quite difficult. Sighted children (wearing blindfolds?) can also take part.

Collect some pieces of cardboard — old cereal packets will do — and a selection of textured fabrics. Place a child's hand on the cardboard and arrange it so that the fingers are together and the thumb slightly apart (mitt shape). Draw round it and cut it out. Repeat the process with the other hand. Use PVA adhesive and stick one pair of mitts to the wrong side of each piece of textured material. Wait for the adhesive to dry, then cut off the surplus material.

During my teaching days I invented this activity for a bright little girl of five who had recently lost her sight. It was important that she should learn to use her fingertips to gather information. Once she could identify the pairs by touch, I expanded the game by putting eyelets in the cuffs of the mitts and showing her how to join the pairs together with

143

treasury tags. This was a useful threading exercise, and probably helped her when it came to learning to insert shoelaces.

FIDDLE TOYS

At every age it seems there are times when we love to 'fiddle' — handling something for the sheer pleasure we receive through our finger tips. Imagine sitting on a sunny beach sifting the dry sand through your fingers, or fiddling with an elastic band. I suppose even stroking the cat might sometimes be considered a 'fiddle'! Activities like these are relaxing and a pleasant tactile experience. Children are inveterate fiddlers, and usually find their own favourite objects. Some children with very special needs may not be able to choose for themselves and might appreciate a ready-made fiddle toy. Here are some suggestions.

A Serendipity of Fiddle Toys

Almost Instant — just allow a little time to collect them all!

Dr Lili Nielson, Danish expert on the education of visually impaired children.

Lili Nielson has a magic suitcase full of bits and pieces, guaranteed to please any child with a passion for fiddling. With such motivation and busy fingers, plenty of tactile experiences are sure to follow! Lift the lid of the case and you will find . . .

- about four strings of beads and buttons, joined together at one end so that the loose ends form a tassel;
- old bed springs, with the ends bent in and protected with sticky tape;
- a pliable soap saver with little plastic suckers on the reverse side;
- a bunch of real keys on a strong ring, with a wooden tag to dangle them by;
- an embroidery frame with tracing paper stretched tightly over it, making it like a flat little drum;
- an electric toothbrush holder, battery driven and without the brush, to switch on and off, so experiencing the pleasant vibration;

144

- three long strands of material, loosely plaited together, so that small fingers can wiggle between the strands;
- a bunch of Bendy Straws, taped together at the long ends so that the bendy parts at the other end can be twisted about in different directions;
- large buttons on a loop of elastic;
- plenty of rattles and tins to shake.

One can imagine any child saying to itself; 'Just let me get at that lot'!

Tactile Bags

Quick

These are made like beanbags (p. 99), but the contents are chosen for their variety and tactile appeal. Ideally, the covers should be fairly thin, so that the contents are easily felt through the fabric, but can't be seen. The idea is to put at least two articles in each bag, so that the child can separate them out by wiggling them about inside. As usual, select items suitable for the group or child in mind. For children with sharp teeth, it may be necessary to use tougher material. Stitch round the seams several times and be extra fussy about closing the gap once the contents are inside. If, in spite of all your efforts, there is any chance that the bags might possibly be opened, make sure the contents will do no harm if eaten. Here are some possible fillings to start you off.

- A slightly inflated balloon and a ping-pong ball.
- Rice and a few large buttons.
- Two curtain rings and some dried peas.
- Orange pips and a marble.
- A cotton reel, some coins or sponge rubber.

Grab Bags

Instant or Quick

These are just an enlarged and tougher version of the tactile bags above. They are intended to be used by children with an iron grip, and are useful for hanging on many of the toy supports suggested in the section on Making Play Possible (p. 5).

For an instant version, use the strong net bags used to package oranges, onions, etc. Partly fill the net with conkers or acorns, in season, or nuts, or shiny, crunchy plastic packaging from a box of tarts — and there you are!

For the quick version, you might start off with a small tin. Inside put bells from a broken toy, buttons, or a few grains of rice, etc. Glue or tape on the lid and enclose the tin in a bag made from brightly-coloured, very strong fabric. (Upholstery material, deck chair canvas, kite material . . . *see* list on p. 151).

Tactile Tortoise

Long-lasting

This strange animal was first made for a small girl with Cerebral Palsy, and before long it became her favourite toy.

I have made several since the prototype and all have enticed idle fingers to be busy. One particular success story was with a teenager in the hospital school where I then worked. She had severe learning difficulties, poor sight and limited movement in her hands. It was difficult to persuade her to join in any of the activities on offer. She only came to life at meal times! One day, in desperation, I put a tactile tortoise on her knee. It was quite heavy — having been well filled with chopped-up tights (for economy!). For this girl the weight was important for she could not ignore the strange object now resting on her knees. During the sing-song that concluded the afternoon, we noticed that her fingers were beginning to explore all the little cushions on the back of the tortoise. Once she found the tail filled with marbles, that was it!

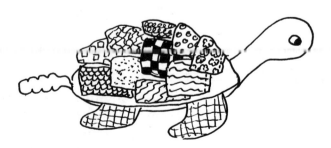

Materials

- Strong material for the body, e.g. tweed, upholstery material.
- Thin material in different colours for the little bags that cover the tortoise's back, and also form the legs and tail.
- Tactile objects to put inside the bags. *See* list on p. 149 . . . for suggestions.
- Scraps of felt for features.
- Stuffing for the head and body. Polyester filling or chopped-up tights.

Method

In the strong material, cut out the underside of the body. Make it oval and about 30 cm (12″) long. Cut out a second oval, slightly larger. This will be humped up to make the curved back of the tortoise.

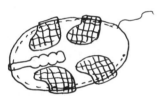

Make several small bags in the thinner material (say eight or ten) and put various tactile objects inside. Arrange the bags on the larger oval (leaving a generous seam allowance round the edge) and machine stitch them in place. (They are supposed to represent the sections of the tortoise's shell!) Make four more bags for the floppy legs and feet (sock shape) and put something tactile in each of them. Tack across the top to prevent the contents from spilling out when you assemble the tortoise. To represent the tail, make a fabric tube. Stretch material is best. Stitch across one end, and put in about four marbles. Leave space between them so that they can be moved about within the tail. Tack across the open end.

Make a neck and head as in the illustration and stuff it firmly. Put this part aside while the rest of the tortoise is assembled. On the *right* side of the underbody pin the legs in position, *facing inwards*. Pin the tail at the back, but make it point towards where the head will be. Gather round the top section of the tortoise, so that it will fit the underbody. Leaving a gap for turning (where the head will go) pin and tack the shell to the underside, making sure the feely parts (shell segments, legs and tail) are tucked inside. Turn the whole thing inside out and you should have a deflated, headless tortoise! Stuff the body firmly, then push the neck into the opening and sew it securely in place with several rounds of ladder stitching. The head makes a convenient handle and will take a lot of strain. If it tends to flop forward, adjust the stitching until it is as you want it.

Bear in mind the tortoise is not easily washed, especially if you have used pasta or rice in the feely bags! It is best kept as a special treasure for an individual child.

Amorphous Beanbag

Quick

Sylvia O'Bryan,
Tutor,
Toymaking

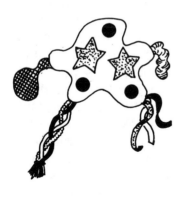

As its name suggests, this beanbag is a wholly unconventional shape. This, of course, is part of its attraction. The body of the beanbag is about the size of a tea plate, but its shape is anything but circular. At two places the material is extended into pairs of 'prongs' which narrow towards their ends and finish with dangling plaits of textured material or bunches of ribbon — lovely to slide between the fingers. The top of the bag is cut slightly larger than the bottom, and a small pocket is inserted roughly in the middle, like the crater of a volcano! This is lined with fur fabric and gathered up with elastic so that an exploring finger can poke around inside. The beanbag is lightly stuffed with dried peas which can be manoeuvred in and out of the 'prongs'. Sylvia obviously has considerable needlework skills, but an Amorphous Beanbag, without the pocket, is no more difficult to make than the conventional and uninteresting (one might even say boring) square or oblong shape. Think of a treasure island with lots of bays and peninsulas and make a beanbag like that. The children will love it!

A Manx Feely Cushion

Quick

This circular cushion, like the emblem for the Isle of Man, has three legs. In this case they are made from small, brightly-coloured socks, each with a tactile or noisemaking object inside, stitched at equal distances round the edge of the cushion. To make it, just cut out two circles of fabric with a pleasant feel, (velvet? fur fabric?) about the size of a dinner plate, and fill three small socks with something tactile

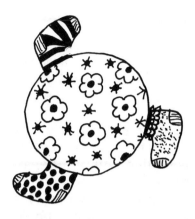

or noisy. (*See* list below and on p. 129 for suggestions.) Tack across the top of the socks to keep the contents inside. Put the circles of material right sides together and arrange the socks (pointing inwards) with their tops at equal intervals around the edges of the circles. Pin and tack them in place. Sew most of the way round the edge of the cushion (twice) leaving a gap for turning and stuffing. Turn the cushion right side out, and stuff the centre with polyester fibre or crunchy paper—or what you will. Close the gap securely.

Suggestions for Contents for Feely Bags

Safety First! Consider carefully the child or children you have in mind before selecting any of the materials on the following list. Something that may be perfectly justifiable and stimulating for one child may be unsuitable—and possibly even dangerous—for another. Some children will always find an inappropriate way of using a toy, and I am sure all readers can think of their own cautionary tales. Vigilance and common sense are the basic essentials for safety, so please use plenty of common sense when selecting from these suggestions. The choice is yours!

Beads—large
Bricks, plastic or wood
Buttons—large
Cotton reels
Crunchy plastic, e.g. packaging tray from a box of
  jam tarts, or paper, e.g. crisp packet
Curtain rings—large
Fish grit
Lolly sticks
Nylon pan scrubber
Plastic shapes from a mosaic, etc
Polyester fibre for a soft feel
Rattle
Rice, etc. (won't wash!)
Real objects, e.g. spoon, comb, tooth-brush, etc.
Shells—large
Smartie tops
Squeaky toy

EXPLORING TEXTURES

Just Feeling

Very quick

Sylvia O'Bryan suggests stitching a soft piece of material (e.g. fur fabric) *inside* a child's pocket. Every time he puts his hand in, he will experience the pleasant texture.

Alison Harland collects together several brightly-coloured pairs of tights, and ties them together to make an exotic octopus. Each leg is stuffed with a different 'feel'. This might be scrunched-up newspaper, plastic foam pipe insulating wrap, ping-pong balls, etc. This wonderful creature can be hung from the ceiling hook, but Alison finds it is more fun to drape it over a couple of children, so that they can play tug-of-war.

Angela Smith (teacher of children with severe learning difficulties) keeps, in her stock cupboard, an extra large bag crammed to the top with tactile objects, ready for the daily 'feely' session. She includes vinyl squeaky toys, soft toys, wooden objects, a small cushion cover filled with plastic packaging, a tin mug — for its cold feel. She saves plastic net bags from the greengrocer and half fills them with pecan nuts, or milkbottle tops, plastic ribbon from the florist, or anything else she thinks will interest the children. She also runs a neat line in the quickest and easiest feely bags it is possible to make! She collects odd socks, puts in a few acorns, or corks, or large buttons — whatever comes to hand — ties a knot in the top of the leg . . . and that is all there is to it.

A Feely Trail Along the Wall

Long-lasting

Seen at a Unit for Young Deaf/Blind Children

This 100% tactile snake wound its way along a corridor wall linking the reception area to the play room. With its help the children could find their way independently from one to the other. It might be an idea worth copying in a domestic situation, where it could be both decorative and helpful in guiding a child from one place to another — even up the stairs — and it would save grubby finger-marks along the wall.

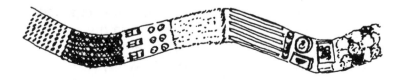

The snake in the unit was made from many pieces of card, (approximately 10 × 20 cm — 4 × 8″) and covered with this imaginative collection of textures:

- Assorted pasta shapes
- Bunches of tissues sprinkled with perfume
- Buttons
- Carpeting
- Cornflakes
- Fur fabric
- Rice
- Sandpaper
- Scotchbrite scourer
- Shiny card
- Strips of macaroni
- Velvet
- Woolly balls

Materials With Tactile Appeal

The following list of suggestions may start you thinking:

Artificial grass — as seen at the greengrocers
Blanket, woolly ordinary weave, or the lanaircell type with holes in
Bubbly plastic — large or small 'bubbles'. Used in packaging and can usually be had for the asking or can be bought at some large stationers and DIY stores
Carpet samples
Chain, metal or plastic, in many sizes. Ironmongers or DIY stores — or garden centres for the plastic kind
Coarse tweed
Corduroy
Felt
Fur fabric, long and short pile
Hessian
Needlecord
Nylon deck chair canvas
Nylon netting, many mesh sizes. Curtaining shops, or garden centres for a strong, large-meshed netting
Nylon pan scrubber, various shapes
Paper in its many forms from tissue to embossed wallpaper or fluted cardboard
Plastic foam from specialist shop or street market
PVC
Prickly doormat
Rug canvas from craft shop
Sand paper, various grades
Satin

Survival blanket from sports shop, in the outdoor
activities section
Taffeta
Terry towelling
Velvet
Vivelle (felt flocked paper from educational suppliers,
p. 4.)

TEXTURE MATCHING

Tactile Cubes

Long-lasting

These feely cubes were created for a small group of
visually impaired children who also had learning
difficulties. I was asked by their teacher to make them
a toy with fairly large tactile surfaces. As it happened,
I was looking for a way to recycle some clean, but
shabby foam bricks. Having just made the colour
blocks on a tray (p. 67), the obvious step seemed to
be to re-cover the foam bricks, using a different texture
for each face. Like the colour blocks, they could be
kept in a shallow box and used for matching and
sorting. Pieces of fur fabric, PVC, velvet, 'bubbly'
plastic (used in packaging), a rough tweed and
corduroy were the textures selected. Then a square
cardboard template was cut, very slightly smaller than
the face of the cube. (If it was the same size, the cover
could turn out to be a sloppy fit, and the cube would
end up a bad shape.) The template was used six times
on each piece of textured fabric. The first square was
drawn, then a gap left for seam allowances before the
second square was marked out . . . and so on, until all
six squares were ready for cutting out. The marking
lines were useful as seam lines when it came to joining
all the squares together. I found the easiest way of
doing this was to lay out all the six piles of different
textures in a line. I took a square from each of the first
two piles and stitched them together, leaving a small
gap at the beginning and end of the seam. (This was
necessary for making an accurate fit when the top and
bottom squares were added.) I repeated the process
until all the squares from the first two piles were paired
together. Then, to each pair, I added a square from
the third pile. To each strip of three I added the fourth

texture. I pinned the ends together, forming a cube without its top or bottom. A square from the fifth pile was sewn to the top of the nearly finished cube, and the process repeated for all the other five. The final squares were stitched to all the bottoms. The pins were removed and the foam bricks forced into their new covers. A knitting needle was useful for persuading them into the corners. The last seams were closed by hand.

In play, the tactile cubes were used in the same way as the colour blocks. The cubes could be turned over within the box until all the faces with the same texture were on top. Fur fabric was the easiest to identify, bubbly plastic the most popular! It did not matter if the children sorted by touch or sight. Once the cubes were correctly arranged, they could run their hands across the top and experience a large area of the same texture. Some learnt to make simple patterns with perhaps two textures arranged alternately as on a chess board, or arranged in rows to make stripes.

Feely Caterpillar

Long-lasting

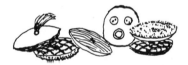

This peculiar creature consists of a series of little cushions joined together with Velcro circles. The back half of one cushion matches in texture the front half of the next, and so the fabrics correspond, domino fashion, all along the caterpillar. The toy is popular with children — I suspect that is because of the ripping sound the Velcro makes!

Materials
- Fabrics with different textures, say six.
- A saucer to use as a template for cutting out the circles.
- A pack of Velcoins — Velcro circles, slightly larger than Velcro Spot-ons.
- A little polyester fibre for stuffing.
- Scraps of felt or buttons for the features.
- A small amount of wool for the tail. (Yes, *this* caterpillar has one!)

Method
Using the saucer as a template, draw two circles on the wrong side of each piece of material. Cut out the circles. Arrange them in pairs, in a row in front of you.

Take a circle from the first pair and give it a face. (Perhaps button eyes and a curtain ring mouth.) Put it back at the head of the row. Take its twin and give it a tassel tail. Put it at the far end of the row. Take a circle from the next pair of textures and sew a Velcoin to the centre. Pin it to the back of the face—wrong sides together for the moment, so that you can see how the sequence of textures works out. Sew the other half of the Velcoin to the matching circle. Back it with a circle from the next pair (Velcoin attached). Continue in this way, matching texture to texture until you reach the tail. The sequence of textures should be perfect, (AB:BC:CD:D . . . A). At this stage it is sensible to check that the Velcro coupling also works, and that you have not inadvertently put two of the same kind on one segment of the caterpillar.

Now to make up the caterpillar. Start with the head. Remove the pins, put the right sides together, tack and sew most of the way round, leaving a gap for turning and stuffing. Turn, lightly stuff and close the gap. Continue like this all down the line of cushions. Velcro them together as you go to check that all is well.

EXPLORING SHAPES

A Tactile Corner

Instant

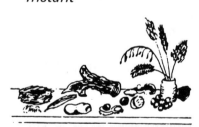

A low shelf or window ledge, set aside for a display of tactile objects, might start off as a fun collection where the family can have its attention drawn to interesting or unusual things. If a child develops an interest in the objects on display, it could possibly turn into a collector's corner or mini-museum. Whatever the outcome, it is worth a try for its obvious educational value. Articles of wood, metal, fur, or plastic could all find a place, but best of all would be things found by (or with) the child such as conkers, acorns, feathers, strange stones . . .

Feely boxes

Feely boxes seem to appeal to every child who is at the right age to appreciate uncertainty and surprise. In my youth, the bran tub at the village fête was always

154

surrounded by a group of children eager to fish around in the bran and see what they could find. Bran tubs, with their special smell, seem to have been replaced with lucky dips, which are often no more than a bucket full of colourfully-wrapped little bundles. Less messy, no doubt, but the presents are not *hidden*, so they completely miss out on the mystery and excitement of the old bran tub. Never mind. These feely boxes can help to redress the balance as children grope inside to make their choice by feel and not by sight.

An Instant Feely Box

Nina Hanson,
Humberside Toy Libraries

Use a strong cardboard box. (The kind that holds whisky bottles is ideal!) Put this in an old stretch nylon cushion cover. The elasticated opening will gather nicely round the top, leaving a hole to dip into.

Another Carton Feely Box

Very Quick

Nursery Nurses,
Bedelsford School

If the carton has flaps for a lid, turn it upside down (flaps now at the bottom). Cut two holes in the new top, fairly near to one side, i.e. not in the centre. These are for the child's arms to reach into the box. On the opposite side, where you will sit, cut a door flap, so that you can secretly change the items in the box. You are now ready for action. A child puts his arms through the holes in the top, you lift the flap and maybe pop in a square brick. When this has been successfully identified, change it for a ball or a soft toy. If the feely box is to be used often, it might be worthwhile decorating the sides with wrapping paper or a collage of old Christmas cards. It is best not to decorate the top. Pictures here could distract the child from the job in hand — which is thinking about the object he is examining by touch.

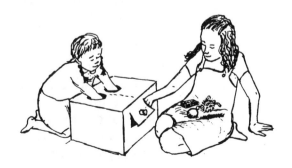

PLAY HELPS

A Smaller
Feely Box

Quick

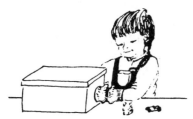

As a Home Tutor I made this simple feely box for Garry, a little boy who had been excluded from school for being so disruptive. I hoped it would hold his attention, and at least help him to concentrate on one thing at a time. I cut the foot off a sock, (turning the leg into a tube) and inserted the cut end into a hole made in the end of a shoebox. I flanged it out and stuck it round the edge of the hole. Garry would hide his eyes while I put something in the box. Then, with the lid firmly on, his hand would go through the sock and into the box to try to identify the object inside. Having made his guess, he could withdraw the object and see if he was right. As his skill increased, I would vary the activity by putting two or more objects in the box, and ask him to find the square one, or the one beginning with a particular letter. Garry responded well to this simple feely box. It came in handy as a 'reward' toy, which could be used to finish off a satisfactory session.

TACTILE BOOKS

Rustly Book

Quick

As a toy librarian I was used to searching among all the toys to find just the right one for a particular child, but one day I drew a blank. I needed a plaything for a little girl who had learning difficulties, a hearing loss, was partially sighted and also had difficulty in using her hands. Quite a challenge for a toy librarian! Every toy suggested had either been borrowed several times before, or was unsuitable in some way. Fortunately, her mother discovered a toy I had overlooked, so she did not leave the toy library empty handed. I promised to try to be creative before her next visit.

We needed a toy which combined noise, movement, colour and a pleasant feel. It should also be safe, strong, and washable. Difficult! It so happened the packer had been generous with the bubbly plastic protecting the last lot of toys received at the toy library, so that could make a starting point. Children love this material for its texture, the rustly noise it makes and the joy of popping the 'bubbles'.

156

I used this material to make a bag like a small cushion cover, and put a few large, brightly-coloured buttons inside. The result was attractive, but of limited appeal. It could be shaken about and the buttons would make a clicking sound as they moved inside the bag, but then what! Several more bags were run up on the sewing machine and different fillings were put in each. I now had a collection of flat feely bags that needed organising into some kind of toy. The best idea seemed to be to join them all together along one side, and turn them into a strange kind of book.

At her next visit to the toy library, the little girl was given her special book—now enclosed in an eye-catching cover. We watched her explore it on her own. She scrunched up the pages, flicked them over, peered at the contents, waved the book about and generally showed her appreciation by playing with it for some considerable time. Satisfaction all round!

Self-help Rustly Book

Quick

A book for children must give pleasure, but it should also be informative and thought provoking. The Rustly Book seemed to satisfy the first requirement, but it might be interesting to try extending the idea. The next book could be more like a real one, telling a story or at least indicating a chain of events.

The purpose of the Self-help Rustly Book was to illustrate, in tactile and visual form, the routine of washing, brushing teeth and combing hair. The book had three pages made in bubbly plastic. A face flannel and a soap dish with a lid (containing strongly perfumed soap) were stitched to the first page. (Small holes were drilled in the base of the dish.) On the second were a toothbrush and an empty tube of toothpaste, still with its screw-top lid, which could be removed for the child to smell the remains of the toothpaste. A comb was stitched to the third page and, alongside it, was a strip of ribbon stitched down at both ends. This held slides and bows which could be removed and used to adorn the child's hair.

A Book of Feely Trails

Long-lasting

This cardboard book was made for Tina, a little girl of six who had recently become blind. As her home tutor, it was up to me to show her how to use her fingertips for gathering information. Quite soon she would need this skill when she began to learn Braille. Inspiration eluded me, but then I remembered seeing at an International Conference of Toy Libraries some attractive mazes for children with severe visual impairment. These were mounted as a wall display but, in use, each one could be played with individually. Each maze was made of string, stitched to a backing of felt which was then mounted on stiff cardboard to make a tile measuring about 20 cm (8") square. The string meandered over the surface of the tile, never crossing over itself, but making an interesting pattern — perhaps forming a spiral, or a staircase, or a snake that curved from side to side. One of the features of each maze was that the beginning was indicated by a bead. Trace the string through to the end, and there was a button (like a full stop) to show you the finish. The mazes were attractive and had obviously been well used. Here was the inspiration I needed.

I began the book of feely trails for Tina. First, I needed the pages. Rectangles of sturdy card about A4 size seemed suitable. A visit to the local stationers produced some large split rings with hinges which would be ideal for holding the pages together. I planned to decorate the pages one by one, and gradually form them into a book, keeping the successful ones and learning from my mistakes!

The first page was quickly made from strips of fur fabric, arranged in lines, with the pile running from left to right. As with the mazes above, the starting point was indicated by a bead, and the finish by a button. This plan was followed throughout the book. Page two was a simple curly trail starting at the top left-hand corner and snaking its way down the page to the button at the bottom right-hand corner. It was formed by a line of finely crushed eggshells which would be slightly scratchy to follow and would, I hoped, encourage a light touch. The crushed eggshell was sprinkled on a line of adhesive, like glitter. Page three was the start of a series of string mazes which became more complicated as Tina's skill increased. The split ring binding for the gradually expanding book was a useful way of keeping the pages together. They need not always be in the same order. I could introduce surprise pages and remove the boring ones when the book was too full.

The book of feely trails led on to various tactile books illustrating stories we shared, or 'Guess What?' pages, where Tina had to try to identify what I had stuck to the page — perhaps a hinged card teapot, which she could lift up and smell the teabag underneath. When inspiration failed, I fell back on some geometric shapes cut from sandpaper.

Tactile Story Books with a Magic Touch

Quick

Mary Digby,
Play Specialist,
Moorfields Eye Hospital

On our toy library shelves, you will find a few tactile books with pictures I have made from fabrics with interesting textures. These are fine as far as they go, but I have a feeling they sometimes appeal to the parents more than to the children! Mary Digby found a way to lift the whole idea of a tactile book onto a more child-centred plane. She and her students made books that related to *real life* situations. They were illustrated with *real* things that could be touched, and sometimes smelt, as the story unfolded. Each book contained several pages, and told about a little girl called Jenny who did ordinary things like 'Visiting Granny'. In that particular story, page 1 described her being smartened up for the occasion. Alongside the writing, the page contained a *flannel* and *soap*, *Noddy toothbrush*, *nail-brush* and *comb*. All these were stuck, with Araldite, to the thick cardboard page. In spite of much handling, they are still there!

On page 2 Jenny's mother made her own preparations. She gave Jenny her spectacles to clean while she packed her handbag for the day. She put in her diary, watch, handkerchief, purse with money in it, and a bunch of keys. All these were mounted on the page.

By page 3 she had finished her preparations and taken the rollers out of her hair, put in her hair clips, chosen a necklace to wear and applied her perfume.

Page 4 described Jenny playing with a Bendy Doll while she waited for her mother. During her play, a button fell off her coat.

By page 5 they had arrived at Granny's. They walked

over the pebbles on the path, smelled the lavender bush and examined the sea shells round the door before they rang the bell.

On page 6 Granny noticed the missing button. She found her thimble, needlebook and thread. She took her glasses out of their case and sewed on the button.

Now it was time for lunch, so Jenny laid the table with a knife, fork, spoon and paper plate. She arranged the plastic flowers to put in the middle.

The final page was all about going home. Granny, true to type, gave Jenny some goodbye presents: a balloon, some sweets and a pen.

In another volume, Jenny visited Moorfields Eye Hospital, and she was introduced to the daily routine, the toys on the ward and the games the children liked to play. Further pages showed the toilet articles on the locker, and the equipment used before Jenny went to the operating theatre. Breakfast the next day would include an individual pack of Rice Krispies, a bendy straw and a sachet of tomato ketchup! After details of the morning's treatment, the book ended on a happy note with a picture Bingo board and all the cards to match to it and, of course, the Lucky Bag prize for winning!

Other titles included 'Jenny Goes to a Birthday Party', 'Jenny spends a night at Granny's House', and 'Jenny Goes on Holiday to Hungary'. This last one described in detail the flight and the experience of staying in an hotel.

With all the lumpy articles stuck to each page, these books were obviously very thick. The stout cardboard pages had holes punched in one side and were tied together with string.

BASIC HAND SKILLS

Pulling

Just Pulling

Instant

Christine Cousins,
Educational Psychologist

1. Present the child with a square box of tissues
Use the decorative kind usually found on dressing tables. Let her pull the tissues out one by one, through the hole in the centre of the lid. Collect up the tissues for future use or for a game of tug-of-war with big brother!

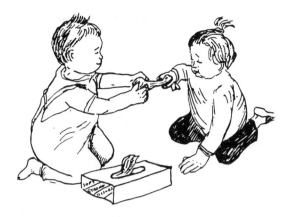

2. Start off with a polythene ice cream container
Make a hole in the lid. String together many strips of thin material. (Make sure the knots will go through the hole in the lid.) Put all the material neatly in the container, thread one end through the hole, put the lid on firmly and invite the child to start pulling. She will be amazed at the seemingly endless string of materials she is producing, and will surely be motivated to carry on to the bitter end. This toy reminds me of the yards of silk handkerchieves magicians can produce from the most unlikely places.

A Spinner

Quick

This is a simple toy that is set in motion by a pulling movement, needing both hands—rather like using a chest expander! It is made from a disc of stiff cardboard (or thin ply) and a length of string, say 1 m (40″) or a little more, depending on the length of the child's arms. Cut out a disc, about 8–10 cm ($3\frac{1}{4}$–4″) in diameter. Rule a line through the centre. On this line make two holes (just large enough to take the string), each about 2 cm ($\frac{3}{4}$″) from the centre. Decorate the disc with a brightly-coloured pattern. Thread the string through both holes and tie the ends together to make a loop. Arrange the disc in the centre of the loop. Hold the loop by both ends and twirl it round to twist up the string. Then move your hands sharply apart to stretch out the string and set the disc spinning. At the critical moment, relax your hands, so that the spinning continues and the string twists round the opposite way. Stretch out again, then relax . . . and so on, to keep

161

the disc spinning. This can take some practice, but it is a fascinating occupation similar to the yo-yo which was all the rage in my childhood.

See also
Jumping Jacks, p. 45
Dancing Danglement, p. 110
Bamboo Mobile, p. 110

Stroking

Children who find it difficult to keep their fingers straight are often encouraged to make a stroking action. Here are two play ways of achieving this movement.

A Furry Caterpillar

Almost Instant

These were all the rage a few years ago, but seem to have disappeared from the shops. They are simplicity itself to make. Just cut a strip of fur fabric about 25 cm (10″) long and 8 cm (3″) wide, making sure the pile runs the length of the strip. The caterpillar rests on your arm, or the upper part of your leg if you are in a wheelchair, with the pile of the fur lying in the direction away from your body. As you stroke the caterpillar along the pile, he will hump himself up in a realistic manner and travel up your arm (or leg!). He can be given character by rounding off his head and tail, and adding eyes and a smiling mouth. Embroider them in wool.

A Paint Sandwich

Quick

This is an alternative to finger painting and considerably less messy! It is a useful alternative when clearing-up time is short. The bread part of the sandwich is made from cling film. A strip of this thin plastic film is spread on the table and a few blobs of finger paint (or powder paint mixed with Gloy adhesive) are dotted here and there. Use different colours for maximum enjoyment. Another layer of cling film is carefully laid on top, avoiding creases and (hopefully) sealing the paint within the sandwich. Using a flat hand, the child can stroke the blobs of paint and spread them out within the sandwich, blending the colours together to make interesting effects.

Note
If the child's hand sticks to the cling film and rucks it up, try resting her palm and outstretched fingers on a pad of fabric.

Squeezing

Here is another hand movement often encouraged by therapists as a way of strengthening a child's grip, and improving his hand function. Everyday living can provide plenty of practice through simple actions like squeezing the water out of the bath sponge or playing with a squeaky toy or playdough, but if you are looking for something a little more sophisticated, try this.

Divers in a bottle

Quick

Daniel Hart,
Student on Work
Experience

I met Daniel when he was working in a Special Class for teenagers with severe learning difficulties. It was a wet day so, at playtime, the pupils were confined to the classroom. Daniel produced his water-filled bottle, complete with two divers, and began to play with it. As he squeezed the sides of the plastic bottle the divers sank gracefully to the bottom. When he stopped squeezing, they bobbed up to the top again. He soon attracted a small group of children, all eager to have a go. For one girl, the fascination of this toy lasted the whole of playtime. She watched her friends play and, when their interest waned, she seized the bottle. She soon discovered how to make the divers plummet to the bottom. Then she began to experiment by placing her hands on different parts of the bottle and applying more, or less, pressure to see how the divers would react.

Materials
- Plastic bottle with cap (e.g. fruit squash bottle).
- Two empty ink cartridges for the divers.
- A small lump of plasticine or Blu-tack.
- Water.

Method
Cut off the pricked ends of the cartridges. Wash them out. Seal the open ends with a blob of plasticine. *Fill* the bottle with water. Insert the divers. Replace the cap.

163

Note

When I copied this excellent toy, I found the amount of plasticine used was critical. Be too generous, and your divers will plunge straight to the bottom. Nothing for it but to empty out all the water and start again! If you do not add enough plasticine, no amount of squeezing will induce the divers to perform. This is why this toy is classified as 'Quick', rather then 'Instant'. Allow a little time for scientific experimentation!

Stacking

Children with poor hand control seldom *choose* to play with a stacking toy. It is difficult and frustrating for them to try to pile one object on top of another, and to place something over a rod may be almost impossible. However, the usual stacking toys on the shop shelves are not the only way of practising this useful skill. Here are some alternatives.

Stack Anything

Instant

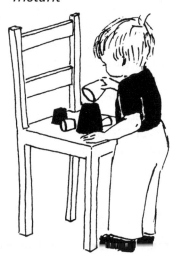

- Christmas cards, the first one opened out as though standing on the mantlepiece, the second one lying horizontally across it, the third one standing on that . . .
- Cotton reels
- Egg-cups
- Flower pots
- Limpet shells—difficult
- Saucepans
- Stones with a flat surface, washed smooth by the sea—painted as an optional extra
- Yoghurt pots or plastic cups

Ideas contributed by Pam Courtney, Christine Cousins and Kanji Watenabi who works with Japanese children.

Higher and Higher

Quick

Lekotek Korea,
The Toy Library,
Seoul

Here is a more conventional stacking toy. It is nothing more than a collection of flat wooden slabs, but it really works! The slabs are made from thick ply or MDF (medium density fibreboard) with all the edges nicely sanded to give a smooth, splinter-free surface. The rectangular slabs are piled up in the usual way but,

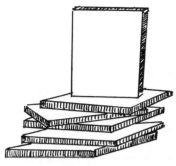

Small, Very Light Bricks

Long-lasting

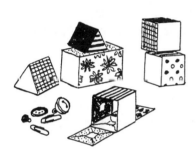

because of their shape, they do not need to be placed precisely on top of each other. A child who cannot manage to stack cube-shaped bricks will have a good chance of success with these. Without being too accurate, it is possible to make a really high tower, giving the child a pleasant glow of achievement. On the way, he will have practised his hand-eye coordination and the skill of grasping and releasing.

Easy to make, but time consuming! These bricks are particularly suitable for 'frail' children. The first set was made for Rupert, a little boy of one-and-a-half, who had Epidermolysis Bullosa. Because of the tender nature of his skin, it was essential for him to have light-weight, washable toys, which would cause the least friction and could be kept hygienic. These bricks can go in the washing machine and wash beautifully at a low temperature.

They are made from squares of plastic cut from a margarine or ice cream tub. Each square is covered with fabric, patchwork fashion, and six are assembled into a cube. Rupert was interested in rattles, so his bricks had either a few foil milk bottle tops, small buttons, paper-clips or a bell inserted. He could use them for stacking, or as a sound discrimination game, grouping together all those with the same contents.

Materials
- Plenty of plastic tubs and boxes. If the plastic is thin and bendy, use it double. There will be a lot of wastage, because only the flat areas are useful.
- Scraps of material. Cotton is best.
- Stiff card or ply for a template; size at your discretion —5 cm square (2″) is suggested. This is too large to be swallowed, but it is a convenient size for small hands.
- Noisemakers if you want your bricks to rattle. Avoid rice, lentils, etc. as these will not wash!

Method
To make one brick
Use the template and cut six squares from the flat parts of the plastic containers. Lay one square onto the

165

material. Cut round it, allowing at least 1 cm seam allowance all round. Fold the top and bottom allowance over the plastic and lace the edges together with a long zigzag tacking stitch. Turn in the other two sides and also zigzag them together, making the corners as neat as possible. Repeat for the other five squares.

Hold two squares together, face to face, and oversew along one edge of the fabric cover. (Make a few extra stitches at the corners for added strength.) Open them out and add two more squares, making a strip of four. Add the two remaining squares, one each side of the strip to make a cross. Fold it up to make a cube. Join together all the unstitched sides by oversewing them, or using ladder stitch. If your brick is intended to rattle, remember to insert the noisemaker before you close the last seam. Make as many more bricks as you need.

Note
It is possible to make these bricks in a variety of shapes, e.g. cut two squares, 5 × 5 cm (2 × 2″) and four rectangles 5 × 5 cm, and you have a double-sized brick. For a ridged roof, cut three squares (or rectangles) and two equilateral triangles, base 5 cm. For a pyramid cut one square and four triangles.

Foam Stacking Bricks

Quick

These are about the size of a house brick, or a little larger. Inside the brightly-coloured fabric covers are blocks of plastic foam, used in upholstery. The plastic foam keeps its shape well. It is also fairly soft, so that a child who finds it hard to pick up a brick in the usual way can handle this set by using a pinching movement and squeezing into the plastic foam. Because of their light weight, they can be handled by children with less than normal strength. Their large size, and the way they can be used to make spectacular structures, makes them attractive to all children who are at the 'stacking stage'.

The plastic foam can be bought, in various thicknesses and density, at specialist shops dealing in upholstery materials and at street markets. It is sold by length and is easy to carve into any size you want. An electric carving knife is the best tool for the job but, failing that, a serrated bread knife will do. Each block of plastic foam is then fitted into an attractive cotton cover. This should be a tight fit so that the finished brick remains a good shape. If you are not too sure how to cover a brick, look back at p. 152.

A Tropical Aquarium

Long-lasting

Mr Poediangga

As a student, Mr Poediangga attended a course at HEARU (Handicap, Education and Aids Research Unit) and invented this clever stacking toy.

Three chunky fish locate over short lengths of dowel fitted into a base board. (For even more stability, this can be clamped to the table.) The thickness of the wood makes the pieces easy to handle and, of course, each fish is attractively painted in brilliant colours.

Materials
- A base board, say 350 × 150 × 20 mm ($14 \times 6 \times \frac{3}{4}''$).
- Three short lengths of dowel, rounded at the top.
- Wood glue.
- A piece of 38 mm ($1\frac{1}{2}''$) soft wood for the fish.
- Paint.
- Polyurethane varnish for protection.

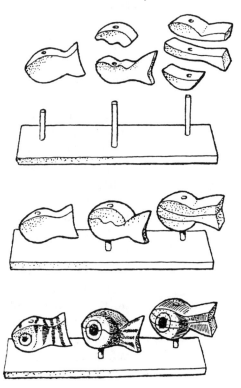

Method

Look at the illustration and drill holes in the base board for the dowel rods. Glue them in place. Cut out the outlines of the fish. Drill a hole through each, slightly larger than the diameter of the dowel for an easy fit. Leave one fish intact, divide the second into two pieces and the last one into three. Sandpaper all the pieces. Paint them as gaudily as possible, then cover with at least two coats of polyurethane varnish.

Now for the ultimate in stacking activities!

Build a Town

Quick

Do you ever organise a festivity for older children where you are fortunate enough to have that rare luxury, plenty of space? If so, the following tale may interest you.

Every year the school for children with learning difficulties where I was then working held a Fun Day. Children, parents and staff all trooped out to the playing field, watched (or took part in) the fancy dress parade, shared a mammoth picnic, then dispersed to the edges of the field to take part in all the activities on offer. Some headed for the candy floss, others fished for plastic ducks in a paddling pool or tried their luck at the hoop-la or lucky dip . . . or whatever else took their fancy.

My contribution to the jollification was to supply a huge quantity of cardboard boxes which had been transformed into giant building bricks. For weeks the senior pupils had been sticking down the flaps and covering the boxes with left-over dregs of emulsion paint donated by staff and parents. The result of all this industry was a huge heap of multicoloured cubes just waiting for someone to build them into something!

As it happened, the first visitor to my patch was a very tall lad. He spent a happy five minutes building a high tower of single boxes. Luckily he realised the biggest should go at the bottom, so managed to achieve a monumental edifice, even taller than himself. It was visible for some distance and soon attracted other would-be builders. Throughout the afternoon, walls, tower blocks, enclosures and 'ruins' were made. All this involved a great deal of thought, bending and

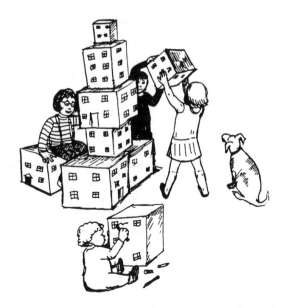

stretching, balancing, etc., but above all, judging by the reactions of both builders and spectators, it helped to put the fun in 'Fun Day'!

Grasp and release

Drop It In

Instant

Pam Courtney,
Teacher of Children
with a Visual Impairment

Pam stores a collection of containers in a large cardboard carton. These include a cake tin, plastic bowls of different sizes, a coffee tin, a wooden box, a plastic ice cream tub, etc. She also keeps handy a variety of objects which can be put into them. She uses plastic and metal spoons, pasta shells, cotton reels, fir cones, stones, woolly balls — anything that can ultimately be sorted into groups. At first the children just put anything into anything! Dropping a metal spoon into a cake tin will make a lovely clatter, and besides being fun, practises the action of grasping and releasing.

A Custom-Made Posting Box

Quick

Peter was a lad with cerebral palsy. Like many other such children, he had great difficulty in letting go of an object once his hands were clasped tightly round it. His Physiotherapist asked me to devise a toy which could encourage him to pick something up, extend his arm, and then release the object. What seemed to be needed was an oversize posting box with only one hole. After a quick survey of all the scrap materials

169

available, a plastic sweet jar was chosen to be the container. This had a wide neck, which made a good target to aim for. The jar was also transparent, so seeing the results of his efforts as he gradually filled it up should give Peter some 'job satisfaction'.

The first problem was how to keep the jar stable, for it was large, and in its empty state very light and easily knocked over. The solution was simple. A few stones were placed in the bottom of the jar and were covered with Polyfilla, mixed to a consistency just sloppy enough to settle between them. When this had set, the jar had a permanently weighted base. Now all that was needed was something suitable to drop into it. Tennis balls were the ideal size to fit Peter's hand but, when using these his jerky movements would scatter them to the four corners of the room. The answer proved to be a generous supply of our old friends, soft woolly balls, stored in a plastic bowl resting on a Dycem mat.

For anyone who missed out on making soft woolly balls in their youth, turn to p. 59 for instructions.

Popper Balls

Quick

Imagine a bag full of a dozen or so brightly-coloured, small felt balls, each fitted with a Velcro coupling, so that they can be linked together, and you will have a mental picture of this toy. The balls are smaller than a tennis ball, but larger than a ping-pong ball —just the right size to fit a small hand comfortably, and for the Velcro to hold them together. The toy library parents who borrow the balls tell me they use them in all sorts of ways. One piles them on her baby's legs for her to kick away, another rolls them over the floor for her son to crawl after, but most say their children like to link the balls together in a long line, or make them into a circle and wear them as a necklace. (There is no danger of strangulation. If the balls are pulled, they simply fall apart.) When creating the toy, I made two balls in each colour so that they could also be used for colour-matching or sequencing. As they are made in felt, they are not washable and sometimes need a trip to the dry cleaners.

Materials
- Felt in several colours.
- Enough Vel-coins for the amount of balls you intend to make. (Vel-coins are circles of Velcro sold in a packet and are slightly larger than Velcro Spot-ons.)
- Polyester fibre for the stuffing.

Method
Each ball is made in six segments, so begin by making a card template. Draw a rectangle about 9 cm × 3 cm ($3\frac{1}{2}'' \times 1\frac{1}{4}''$). Mark the centre of each side with a cross. Draw a petal shape that touches all four crosses and cut it out. To make one ball, draw round the template six times. Cut out the pieces and stitch them together, leaving a gap at one end for the stuffing. Stuff the ball fairly firmly. (It must be easy to grasp, but beware of making it too heavy or the Velcro will have a struggle to hold all the balls together.) Close the gap, and sew one half of a Vel-coin to the North Pole and the other to the South. Repeat the process as many times as necessary.

Peg toys for finer finger movements

The action of putting a peg in a hole helps a child to use 'tripod grip', i.e. holding a peg between thumb and two fingers. This action is often needed in daily life for such simple tasks as picking something up or holding a pen. Some children find this action difficult, and need plenty of practice with motivating toys. These can often be found in toy libraries, so if you have one near you try there first. Otherwise look in the toy shop for Escor Toys (*see* list p. 4 for mail orders) or plastic toys with large play people. (Fisher Price, Little Tykes, etc.) When large pegs can be confidently managed, the time has come to move on to smaller pegs that need a finer finger movement. Here toy manufacturers are not so helpful. Fortunately, medium-sized peg toys are easy to make, if you use wooden dolly pegs as a starting point (*see* Colour Peg Tin, p. 65). Saw off the 'legs' and you are left with a neat little peg man all ready for painting. If you have access to a lathe, it is not difficult to turn your own peg men from dowel, and by making them yourself you can adjust the height if necessary.

The Peg Bus

Long-lasting

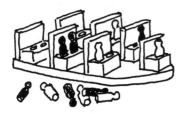

This was originally made in a workshop for adults with learning difficulties. It has been copied many times, and is a firm favourite with the children of three and upwards who come to our toy library. The bus is meant to represent a mini-bus, with the driver in front and the passengers sitting in pairs behind him. The seats have holes drilled in them. These are slightly wider than the pegs and fairly deep to allow the passengers to fit in easily and securely. The pegs are coloured in pairs so that the toy can also be used for colour matching — the two yellow ones sharing the same seat. (The driver wears a white coat.) The bus is not fitted with wheels. This not only simplifies the construction, but prevents the bus from moving just as a peg man might be put in a hole.

Colour Peg Board

Long-lasting

Truncated dolly pegs were also used to make this toy. It does not have such opportunities for imaginative play as the peg bus above, but it had many fans among the class of children with learning difficulties who played with the prototype. A fairly large piece of chipboard made the base. This was divided into squares, and a hole was drilled in the centre of each to take a peg man. Then every square was painted a different colour with a peg man to match.

Note
These pegs can have many more uses, e.g. a child might like to play Snakes and Ladders or Ludo, but has difficulty in manipulating the counters. Perhaps a wooden board with holes in the appropriate places, and peg men to move round it, might solve the problem.

Peg Pictures (Small pegs)

Long-lasting

(For use with children who have passed the stage of putting things in their mouths.) These pictures use brightly-coloured plastic pegs about 2 cm long, sold by Galt and many other educational suppliers

p. 4. Normally they fit into boards which have rows of holes drilled in them, usually 25–100. For some children these are very satisfactory. They enjoy the task of putting a peg in every hole, perhaps filling up a row with all one colour, or designing complicated patterns. For others they have little or no appeal. This is a pity, for placing the tiny pegs in the board is an excellent way of practising fine finger movements and hand-eye coordination! I began experimenting with my own peg boards with holes strategically placed, so the addition of some pegs would complete a picture. As usual, one idea led to another.

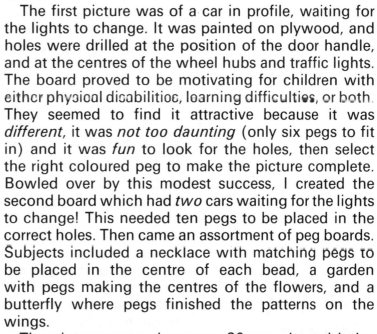

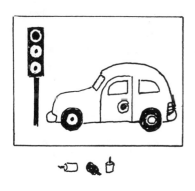

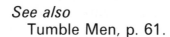

The first picture was of a car in profile, waiting for the lights to change. It was painted on plywood, and holes were drilled at the position of the door handle, and at the centres of the wheel hubs and traffic lights. The board proved to be motivating for children with either physical disabilities, learning difficulties, or both. They seemed to find it attractive because it was *different*, it was *not too daunting* (only six pegs to fit in) and it was *fun* to look for the holes, then select the right coloured peg to make the picture complete. Bowled over by this modest success, I created the second board which had *two* cars waiting for the lights to change! This needed ten pegs to be placed in the correct holes. Then came an assortment of peg boards. Subjects included a necklace with matching pegs to be placed in the centre of each bead, a garden with pegs making the centres of the flowers, and a butterfly where pegs finished the patterns on the wings.

The pictures were drawn on 20 mm ply and holes were drilled at the appropriate places. These were large enough for the little plastic pegs to fit in comfortably. The picture was painted, and protected with two coats of polyurethane varnish. The matching pegs were stored in a film spool container and kept in a net curtain bag, together with the board.

See also
Tumble Men, p. 61.

Posting

A Simple Posting Box with Only One Hole

Instant

This toy can be a winner for any child who is just starting to take an interest in putting one thing inside another. This can happen at any age from about ten months upwards. As well as being good fun, cheap, and easy to make, this simple posting box makes a good introduction to more complicated commercial ones.

All you need is a tin with a plastic lid and a supply of cotton reels to post inside. The tin should be as large as possible. Make sure the lip is 'rolled' (not sharp) and that the cotton reels are all the same size. Use one as a template to mark a circle in the centre of the lid. Cut this out — with scissors, or with a heated needle embedded in a cork so that you can hold it comfortably. The hole should be slightly larger than the reel so that it will drop through easily. Check there are no jagged edges to the circle. (A rub with sandpaper will remove them.)

To make this simple toy more attractive, paint the tin and reels with Humbrol enamel. One coat should be sufficient, and you will end up with an attractive and colourful toy with twice the child appeal.

At the Sense Centre (for deaf/blind children) the teachers use a series of simple one hole posting boxes. They consider the special needs of the children with flaccid hands. The hole in the lid is made slightly smaller than the object to be posted, so that pushing it through the hole requires some effort. The children begin with a ping-pong ball. When they are successful, the ping-pong ball falls into the tin with a satisfying clonk. As they become adept at this, they move on to another tin with a smaller hole which will just accept a wooden bead. Next comes a third for posting plastic hair curlers. These present a new problem. They need to be up-ended before they will fit into the hole. The sound and feel of the little plastic bristles on the sides of the curlers rubbing against the edge of the hole can set the teeth of an adult on edge but, of course, the children love it!

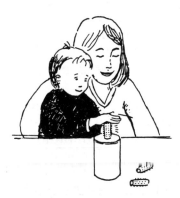

Posting Acorns in a Bottle

Instant

Susan Myatt,
Parent,
Kingston-upon-Thames
Toy Library

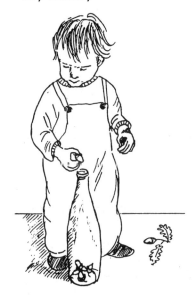

All children love to play with natural objects and things from the adult world. These are the nuts and bolts of our environment, and through them children learn about the world in which they live. Picture in your mind's eye a two-year-old totally absorbed in fitting the lids on heavy saucepans. A year later, he may be splashing in the puddles or scuffing up the Autumn leaves, while at home his big sister is playing at weddings, draping herself in an old net curtain and wearing her mother's shoes. Some children cannot share in these delights, but *if* you are reading this in the Autumn, and *if* you live near an oak tree, and *if* your child has reached the 'posting' stage, here is a chance to bring the outside world nearer to him, and let him practise his new-found skill into the bargain — and all completely free!

All you need is a bag full of acorns (perhaps you can collect them together) and a plastic bottle. If you want your child to practice fine finger movements, choose a bottle with a neck just wide enough to accept an acorn on end. Now sit back and watch his delight as he sees the bottle gradually filling up because of his own skilful efforts.

Posting Drinking Straws in a Bottle

Instant

Lorraine Crawford's
little daughter

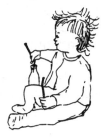

This idea is similar to the one above, but it has two advantages. It can be set up in seconds, so really is 'instant', and it does not rely on a seasonal crop of acorns.

Lorraine's small daughter was playing on the kitchen floor when an empty milk bottle caught her attention. Here was an unusual container just waiting to be filled! She tried to push a spoon down the neck, but in spite of all her efforts, the bowl remained outside. She searched around for something else to try. She had instant success with a pot of pencils, but even better was a bunch of drinking straws someone thoughtfully provided. These were long and bendy, and needed to be lined up with the neck of the bottle before they could be dropped inside.

Threading

Threading is a peaceful activity with many useful spin-offs. It encourages the use of both hands as well as hand-eye coordination. Other skills, such as colour matching, sorting or grading, can also become part of it. Leaving aside all these worthy attributes, most children at some stage in their lives really *enjoy* threading beads!

First of all, the skill of poking the threader through the hole must be learnt.

- In an Australian toy library the children begin by threading large haircurlers onto a length of plastic pipe.
- At Lekotek Korea, they use blocks of wood with holes bored through them and a piece of dowel to use as a threader. As the child's skill increases, bricks with smaller holes are provided.
- At some toy libraries in the UK, the children follow Roy McConkey's suggestion and thread plastic rings, cut from a washing-up liquid bottle, over a broom handle.
- Threading toys are, of course, available from toy shops. One is a set of plastic leaves with holes in them. By using the threaders provided, the veins on the leaves can be outlined. There are more ideas in the educational catalogues listed on p. 4 or here is a threading toy you can make yourself.

The Bee in a Tree

Long-lasting

This delightful threading toy first appeared in the 'Making Toys' programme televised by the BBC in 1975. Its designer, David Chisnell, created a plywood tree shape, which had several holes drilled in the leafy part. A length of cord was tied to the tree trunk, and on the other end was a busy bee made from a short length of dowel. The bee could 'fly' in and out of the holes until all the string was used up. This toy had a practical feature. The bee was attached to it, so could not be dropped or lost!

Materials

Either

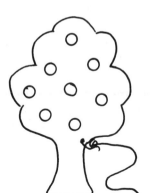

- an old table tennis bat with the rubber face removed, *or*
  a small piece of good quality ply, 5 mm or 7 mm, for the tree.
- About 5 cm (2") of dowel for the bee, (longer rather than shorter) or you could use a long, fat macrame bead.
- A length of thin cord, say 20–30 cm (8–12") or longer, depending on how far the child in question can stretch. Blind cord is best. This will not kink.
- An electric saw or fretsaw.
- A large drill for making holes for the bee to fly through, and a very small one for the hole in the back of the bee and for attaching the cord to the tree.
- A dab of strong adhesive and a matchstick (for fixing the cord in the hole in the bee.)
- Sandpaper.
- Paint, and polyurethane varnish for protection.

Method

Draw a tree shape on the plywood as suggested in the illustration. Shape out the bottom of the tree trunk to make it easier to grasp. Cut out the tree. Drill holes at intervals in the leafy part. Drill a small hole in the trunk for the cord. Clean up all the rough edges with sandpaper. Round off the ends of the dowel (with sandpaper) and drill a small hole in one end to take the cord. Paint both sides of the tree green, with a brown trunk. Paint the bee yellow with black stripes. Protect all the paint with two coats of polyurethane varnish. Tie one end of the cord to the tree. Squirt some glue into the hole in the bee and poke in the other end of the cord. A needle is helpful to feed it in. Wedge it firmly in place with a small piece of matchstick coated with glue.

The Happy Tree

Long-lasting

This is a more complicated threading toy than the one above. The holes are much smaller, and are arranged in pairs. Birds, or butterflies, or fruit are attached to the tree by threading them in position. The loaded tree

177

looks rather like a jolly version of a William Morris design! It was given its name by a young user who was attracted by the bright colours of the adornments. If there are plenty of pieces of each shape, a child can change the appearance of the tree as he pleases. One day a flock of birds might roost in it, and another time butterflies might settle there. Perhaps it is Autumn and the apples are ripe!

Instructions are given for the felt version which, because of its size and light weight, is particularly suitable for some frail children. The tree is equally attractive and more easily washed when made in wood in the same way as the tree above.

Materials

- Felt — green and brown for the tree, and small scraps of bright colours for the adornments.
- A leather punch.
- Eyelets — used for reinforcing holes in belts, etc. Obtainable from craft shops. The tool for their application is included in the pack. Provide your own hammer!
- Stiffening — buckram, pelmet lining or heavy duty Vilene.
- A narrow, round shoelace. Look for a pair with long tags on the ends.

Method

Make a paper pattern. Fold a sheet of paper in half. Draw half the tree up to the fold line, cut out the shape and open up the paper. If you are satisfied with your tree, use it as a pattern — if not, try again! Place the pattern on the green felt and draw round the leafy part of the tree twice. Cut out both shapes. Repeat the process on the brown felt for the trunk. Cut out the *whole* tree from the stiffening material. Sandwich this between the layers of felt and oversew or blanket stitch all round the edge. Punch holes in pairs in the leafy part of the tree. Measure the distance between them carefully. It must be exactly the same for every pair, for the holes in the tree must match up accurately with the holes in the adornments.

Next make the adornments. Trace off a bird or

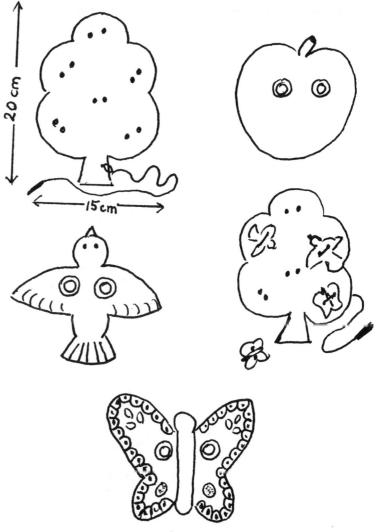

Actual size

butterfly from the illustrations, and cut them out
in double felt. Decorate the top shape with a few
embroidery stitches — eyes and feathers on the birds,
spots on the wings of the butterflies. Stitch the two
parts together (oversew or blanket stitch round the
edge), and accurately punch a pair of holes in each,
so that they will exactly match up with the holes on
the tree. Reinforce *all* the holes with eyelets. Attach a
threader to the trunk of the tree. Finally, provide a box
or bag to keep the tree and all its adornments clean
and together.

Making a Necklace

It takes a steady hand to hold a bead in position and aim a threader through the hole in the middle. Avoid the frustration (and possible bad temper) that can happen if beads roll out of reach, or the threader will not go through the hole easily. Here are some tips to consider.

1. Provide a container for the beads. A plastic cereal bowl is ideal. If keeping it upright or in one place is a problem, fix it to the table with a blob of Blu-tac, or a loop of masking tape.

2. Make sure the threader will go right through the bead and out the other side. Sometimes a round shoelace will do the job, but large beads may need a special threader available from educational suppliers. Nearer to hand is the polypropylene clothes line — the thin one without a wire core, used for whirly lines. This goes through the large holes in wooden beads very successfully, and is stiff enough to come well out of the hole for easy grasping and pulling through. Jewellers sell nylon threaders with a stiff wire end, which are excellent for older children who wish to thread small beads.

3. Brightly-coloured wooden beads can be bought at most toy shops. Square ones will not roll away and are easier to hold than round ones which can easily slip through the fingers. Attractive adult beads which appeal to older children can often be bought at car boot sales, etc.

Threading for Children with Poor Hand Control

Quick

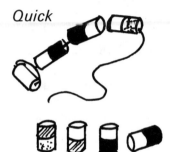

My favourite first 'beads' are made from the cardboard or plastic tubes that come from the till rolls in supermarkets. These are about 5–7 cm long (2–$2\frac{3}{4}''$) and have a very large — almost impossible to miss — hole down the centre. Ask nicely and the checkout staff will be delighted to save them for you.

Suitably painted in bright colours and given a protective coat of polyurethane varnish, they can look very attractive. Use polypropylene clothes line mentioned above as a threader.

For tactile threading, use these same till rolls and simply substitute textured fabric for colours.

**Making Your
Own Beads**

178

Small Light Beads

Long-lasting

1. *Threading on a Pipe-Cleaner*

This is an 'instant' activity which delighted my own children one boring wet day many years ago. It has intrigued Kingston Toy Library children at intervals ever since! It is for children with nimble fingers.

Cut a few plastic drinking straws into short lengths and put them on a saucer or dish so that they are easier to pick up and do not roll all over the table. Give out the pipe-cleaners, and let the children thread the pieces of straws onto them to make bracelets for themselves or necklaces for dolls or teddy bears.

2. *Making Paper Beads*

These have been around for so long that they might even be considered traditional. Some parents of my generation may have forgotten to pass on this absorbing activity, so here it is. The beads are made by rolling up strips of paper. All you need is a knitting needle, (the larger the size, the bigger the hole in the middle will be), any non-shiny paper, some PVA adhesive, and some paint or felt pens for decorating the finished beads.

Suppose you choose to use newspaper. Tear it against the edge of the table, or a ruler, into strips say 24 × 5 cm (10 × 2″). Take one strip and start to wind it round the knitting needle. Then paste the strip and continue to wind it round, forming a cylinder. Slide it off the needle and put it to one side to dry. It is best to wind near the tip of the needle so that the bead will slip off easily. Avoid putting adhesive on the needle. When you have become skilful in rolling these beads, you might try larger or smaller ones or even give them a rounded shape by using strips of paper that taper off like a pennant.

If you use wall paper, the beads will turn out chunkier, and you will need a shorter strip. Once the adhesive is dry, the beads can be decorated.

These unusual beads are made from short lengths of bamboo. They are very light in weight, yet have a fairly large hole through the middle. These features make them specially suitable for 'frail' children, and for others who might benefit from using their fingers in a threading action. Each bead is individually painted so, into the bargain, they can string up into an attractive necklace, which is likely to make the wearer the envy of all her friends!

Materials
- Some fairly sturdy bamboo garden canes — say two, but it depends on how many beads you wish to make.
- A craft knife.
- A knitting needle.
- Sandpaper.
- Paint: acrylic is best, poster will do.
- Polyurethane varnish.
- A threader, and a box to hold the beads.

Method
Remove the waxy layer from the outside of the bamboo with a craft knife. (Scrape away from yourself.) Cut the bamboo into lengths of about $2\frac{1}{2}$ cm (1"), avoiding the joints and any uneven parts. Clean out the pith from the centre with a knitting needle. Rub each bead with sandpaper to make a really smooth surface. Now for the fun part! Decorate each bead with a pattern, or tiny flowers, or as your fancy dictates. Protect each bead with polyurethane varnish and put them in a box, complete with threader. A set of hand crafted beads like these can make a very special and unusual present.

Paper tearing

Perhaps one of the most blissful moments in the life of my toddler son was when he was given an old telephone directory and full permission to let rip! The physical action of tearing paper is infinitely satisfactory to a small child at the 'destruction' stage. Of course, this abandoned paper tearing must not go unchecked once a child starts to use books 'for real', but even then, paper tearing can be given a mask of respectability if it is indulged in for a creative purpose.

In many schools the children learn to tear shapes,

182

starting with squares and triangles, progressing on to curves like a circle or a crescent moon. Then they are ready to tear the shapes for collage pictures. These are sometimes done in silhouette, and can look very effective when the slightly rough edge of the torn black shape is pasted onto a white background.

Making a neat tear in a sheet of paper calls for both hands to be carefully controlled. A satisfactory tear will be more likely if the child holds the paper close to the line he will be tearing, thumbs touching. Then he should work slowly, making small movements for each tear.

Now for a paper tearing exercise which results in an aeronautical toy guaranteed to intrigue a child — and any grown-ups who happen to be around.

A Helicopter

Instant

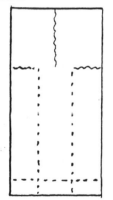

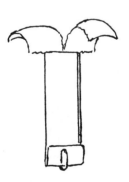

If your child is already a confident paper tearer, he can have a go at this. If he is not yet quite skilful enough for the fairly careful tearing required, try making it for him. At least, it makes a splendid tracking toy. At most, it might spur him on to try again.

You need a rectangle of paper, say cheap notepaper, not too thick, about 10 × 20 cm (4 × 8″). About a third of the way down one side, make a tear a third of the distance across and fold in the longer section. (Your paper now vaguely resembles a garden spade!) Turn up the bottom and crease across firmly. A paper clip will keep it in place and add a little weight. To make the 'rotor blades' tear down from the middle of the top edge as far as the folded part. Bend one blade towards you and the other away from you. Give them both a slight curve as in the illustration. Now for the maiden flight! Hold the helicopter up high, let go, and watch it spiral its way towards the floor — in the manner of a sycamore seed.

Note
Watch which way your helicopter turns — clockwise or anti-clockwise? Bend the rotor blades in the opposite direction, and now see what happens!

Paper cutting

There is something very satisfying about the action of snipping with scissors — the noise perhaps, or the feel. Most children seem to enjoy using scissors, but for some the physical action of bringing the blades together can be difficult, and the best they might achieve could be a straight snip.

First, let us consider the scissors. There is a choice of several different types of special ones for children, available from educational suppliers (p. 4). Some are designed to be used by the child with an adult hand covering his — and really doing most of the work! This helps the child to learn the opening and closing action needed to manipulate the blades. Perhaps the more popular scissors are the self-opening kind that have had the finger and thumb rings on the handle removed. These are replaced by a strip of springy plastic which covers one handle, then curves over to cover the other, joining them together with a pliable loop. The handles of the scissors are compressed in the normal way, and the loop is flattened. When the child stops squeezing, the handles spring apart, automatically preparing the blades for the next cut.

Assuming we now have our mythical child happily snipping with his new scissors, how can we provide an outlet for this new-found skill? Some of the following suggestions only require a straight snip, others need more careful scissor control. It is always possible to compromise, with the child doing the snipping bits and leaving the accurate cutting to you.

1. *Make a garden picture*. Your child snips green paper to represent grass. You cut out flowers (from old seed catalogues?) and together you assemble your efforts on a backing sheet.
2. *Make a mosaic picture*. Think of an ancient Roman floor with its hundreds of tiny squares and triangles arranged in an elaborate design. Perhaps such pattern making is not for you, but a child can achieve a similar effect by snipping shapes and arranging them so that they overlap and cover a specific area — perhaps the shape

TOUCH

of a tree or a flower. Supposing she decides to make a blue flower. Look together in old magazines for advertisements with lots of blue on them, sea or sky perhaps. Draw the flower while she snips up the blue parts of the pictures —pieces not too small if she wants a quick result! Then the pieces are stuck within the outline of the flower, and the outcome should be a pretty mosaic blossom and a child with an increased ability to snip.

3. *Making a waver.* Start with a short length of dowel for the handle. Then your child snips up plenty of long strips of paper. Stick these to the end of the handle and bind them in place with string or wool. The waver can be shaken to make a rustling sound, or moved about in time to music in similar fashion to the huge pom-poms used by cheer leaders at an American ball game!

4. *Make some paper lanterns* to add to the decorations at party time. Use wrapping paper, or plain paper, child-decorated with a pattern. For each lantern, cut the paper into a rectangle, about A4 size. Cut a strip off one end, say 2 cm ($\frac{3}{4}''$) wide, to be the handle of the finished lantern, and put it to one side. Fold the paper in half, long sides together. Cut into the folded edge and stop just over half way across. Make the cuts the whole way along the folded edge. Open out the paper and stick the short sides together, overlapping them slightly, to make a cylinder. Gently press on the top to push the fold slightly outwards and increase the gaps between the cuts. Retrieve the handle and stick it in place.

   Tiny lanterns made this way in foil paper come in handy as Christmas tree decorations.

5. *Make a convection snake.* Start with a circle of cartridge paper about the size of a tea plate. Beginning at the outside edge, start cutting a strip that widens out to be about $1\frac{1}{2}$ cm (just over $\frac{1}{2}''$) across, and spirals its way towards the centre like the grooves in a gramophone record. You should finish up in the centre with a blob

shape like a snake's head. Make a continuous pattern on both sides of the snake. Tie a knot on the end of a length of thread and pass the other end through the snake's head. Hang it over a radiator where the rising hot air will make it twist on the end of the thread. Alternatively, stick a pencil in a cotton reel base and rest the snake's head on the point. Put it on the shelf above a radiator.

It takes considerable skill to cut out a respectable spiral. Most beginners appreciate a line drawn for them to follow.

6. *An out-of-date mail order catalogue has many potential uses.* Full length pictures of people can be cut out to make paper dollies and arranged in families, or a class of children at school. Furniture and household goods can be cut out and stuck in the appropriate places on a large picture of a section through a house — beds in the bedroom, pots and pans in the kitchen, etc.

7. *Old Christmas cards* are wonderful for cutting up. They can be used to make a counting book — one Christmas tree, two snowmen, etc. — and, of course, to make a scrapbook. When Mary Digby was the Play Specialist at Moorfields Eye Hospital, she made tiny scrapbooks which the children could fill at one sitting. Parents or older children cut out the scraps for the little ones, who could pick out their chosen pictures from a box, and stick them in their books with Pritt Stick adhesive.

8. *Silly pictures.* I know one group of children with learning difficulties where the joke is to cut out and paste together silly pictures, e.g. someone might cut out a kitchen and stick a horse in the middle of it or a man might wear a wheelbarrow on his head. The possibilities are endless and all good for a laugh!

See also
Christmas Cards, p. 86.

BUTTONS, BOWS, AND POPPERS

Buttons

Scenes and Faces

Long-lasting

Monica Taylor,
Toy Librarian,
The Rix Toy Library

Monica makes colourful and motivating pictures where buttons play an essential part in the design. They may be needed to attach separate items to a picture or they might be used to complete a face. The pictures can be played with on the floor or table. With all the pieces in place, the larger ones hang on the wall as an attractive decoration. She has found them particularly useful for a little group of children with Down's Syndrome, but they are so colourful and attractive that everyone wants to have a go.

Supposing Monica wants to make a country scene. She will start with a background of calico and stitch to this a tree, a hill and some grass, cut from felt or any suitable material. Next, she attaches buttons (perhaps of different sizes) in strategic places, ready to receive the colourful felt shapes—each with a button hole—which will bring the picture to life. These are all made in felt, reinforced and stiffened with iron-on Vilene, and could be in the shape of birds, butterflies or apples to attach to the tree, or perhaps some rabbits and flowers for the grassy hill.

The faces, human or animal, are made slightly differently. Monica cuts two layers of fabric, face-shaped, and stitches them together at the top. On the top layer she makes button holes in the right position for the eyes, nose and mouth and adds hair, ears, whiskers, etc. as appropriate. On the bottom layer she

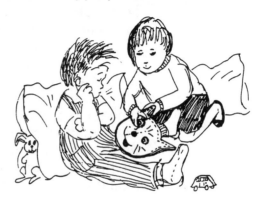

stitches suitable buttons to be threaded through the holes and so complete the face.

Inspired by Monica, I have also tried my hand at button pictures. These began as a series of button trainers I made for children with learning difficulties. At first they were like a simple rag book with only two pages, similar to Monica's button faces, turned on their sides. The buttons were stitched to the second page, and were threaded through the first. This idea was quite successful. There were no loose parts to be lost but, as I increased the number of buttons on the second page, it became obvious that the ones near the spine were quite difficult to manipulate. To overcome the problem, I made the next button trainer circular in shape. Using a dinner plate as a template, I cut two circles of fabric, and joined them together with a small circle of stitches in the centre. The most attractive buttons I could find were stitched to the unattached part of the bottom circle, and could be easily threaded through the holes in the top one. The button circle was all very well in its way, but like my button books, I felt it was *boring*! It reminded me of a plate shape—after all that was its origin!—so I thought of a way of adding some food. I used some odd scraps of ply to cut out 'buttons' representing a full English breakfast! Now a fried egg, sausages, mushrooms, tomatoes, and bacon could all be threaded through their respective holes to fill the plate!

Car Button Trainer

Long-lasting

On the same principle of two pages, buttons on the second, a picture on the first, I have made a button trainer which has found favour with many of the toy library children. On the first page is a stitched picture of a child sitting in a car, waiting for the lights to change. Attached to the second page are the buttons for the wheels, the steering wheel, the car door (which opens) and the traffic lights. This simple scene seems to motivate even the most reluctant 'buttoners'! Every time the picture is given to a child—with the buttons not threaded through—their fingers get busy. In no time the car is complete with its wheels in place, and all the other buttons soon follow suit. It has well repaid the two evenings it took to make.

Button Snake

Long-lasting

This peculiar reptile is just a series of cloth segments, reducing in size from head to tail, each buttoning to the one in front. As the buttons are arranged in pairs, the segments are easy to link up in the right order.

Materials
- Buttons — number of pairs and size according to the ability of the children.
- Fabric, for top pieces and linings.
- Button thread.
- Card or paper for a pattern.

Method
Draw patterns for the segments, the largest (i.e. for the head and following segment) about 10×14 cm ($4 \times 5\frac{1}{2}''$). Make the pattern for the next segment about $1\frac{1}{2}$ cm narrower and shorter, and so on all down the line. Put the patterns on the wrong side of the fabric and draw round them. Cut *outside* the pencil lines. (They come in handy later as a stitching guide.) Round off the head and tail. Lay all the components out in front of you — top pieces, linings and pairs of buttons. You will see from the illustration that the head and tail have only one button each. All the other segments have two — the first to button to the segment ahead and the second (a dummy) to match the one that

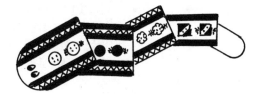

follows. Sew all the buttons to the top pieces. Then, beginning with the head, sew the top piece to its lining by putting right sides together, stitching most of the way round. Turn it right side out and close the opening. (Top stitch or oversew.) Make the buttonhole. Repeat the process all the way down the snake, remembering to adjust the size of the button hole as appropriate.

189

A Train with Button Couplings

Long-lasting

The special feature of this train, which appears on the cover, is that the engine and carriages link together with toggles and loops, which are the fastenings used on a duffle coat. Young children find it hard to manipulate these fastenings while the coat is on their back, because they can't see what their fingers are doing. The coupling together of the train provides a good example of learning through play. A child who can poke a toggle through a loop is well on the way to pushing a button through a slot.

The train is made from plastic canvas and covered overall with brightly-coloured wool stitches. The carriages, or trucks, are open (as in the early days of railways), so can be filled and emptied as the child's play requires. The train is washable, light in weight, and can have as many carriages as your enthusiasm allows. The directions may seem daunting, because I have tried to describe each operation in detail, but once you have grasped the principle you can do it your way! The end result will be well worth the effort.

Materials

- One sheet of 7 mesh plastic canvas.
- Double knitting wool in several bright colours, and a scrap of black for the funnel.
- Buttons for the wheels — four for each vehicle.
- Toggles — one for each carriage, and one for the engine if it is likely to do any shunting. Otherwise a towing loop is sufficient.
- Piping cord for the loops. Say size 4.
- The lining of the trucks and engine is optional, but it makes them even stronger and looks good! It needs thin card, some thinnish fabric — like cotton, and strong glue.

Method

To make one truck. Cut out the base, making it 16 holes (17 bars) × 26 holes (27 bars). Thread a length of piping cord (say 12 cm — 6″) through the toggle and back on itself. Sew the ends of the cord firmly to the base, stitching through the plastic canvas, but stopping just short of the edge, or the piping cord will be in the way when you come to put the truck together. The

Side of trucks

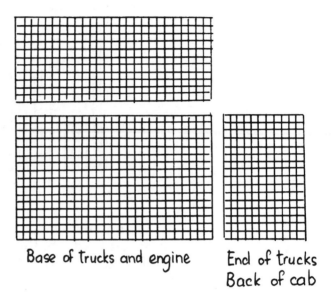

Base of trucks and engine   End of trucks
                             Back of cab

toggle should stick out in front about $2\frac{1}{2}$ cm (1"). Stitch a loop of piping cord to the other end of the base, again stopping just short of the edge of the plastic. Make sure the loop is large enough to accept a toggle fairly easily. Put the base to one side. Next cut out the sides, 26 × 11 holes. Cut out the two ends, 16 holes × 11 holes. Using double wool, cover these four pieces with tapestry stitch or tent stitch, — both cover the canvas well — oversew the sides and ends together. Now return to the base. Oversew the top of the truck to the base, making sure the piping cord is underneath or the top will not fit on properly. Add some extra stitches at the corners as necessary. Attach the button wheels, so that the bottom of the rim lies just below the base of the truck. This is a fiddly job, but has to be done at this stage. If they are attached to the base before the truck is put together, it is impossible to oversew behind them. Neaten the top of the truck by oversewing all round it, again making extra stitches at the corners as necessary.

If you decide to line the truck, cut card rectangles to size, cover them with fabric (stick or stitch) and stick them in place.

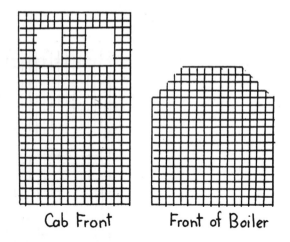

Cab Front   Front of Boiler

The engine is made by the same method. Cut out the base and attach the loop and toggle? as before. Follow the diagram for the dimensions of the other pieces. Cut them out. (The front of the cab, with windows, is cut twice, making this section double thickness. This will give it rigidity.) The two front sections of the cab are not needed until later, so ignore them for the moment. Cover all the other pieces with stitching, then put the back of the cab to one side. (Without this in place, it is easier to attach the funnel and the wheels when the time comes.) Oversew the boiler to the curved front, bending the boiler to shape as you go and making sure the corners meet at the bottom. Now make the funnel. Cut a strip of canvas, say 8 × 22 holes — this allows for an overlap. Starting about two holes in, cover most of the strip with black wool. When you nearly reach the edge, overlap the ends and sew through both layers of canvas. Oversew the raw edge at the top and the bar still visible at the side. Stitch the funnel to the centre of the boiler. Oversew the (part-finished) engine to the base. Attach the wheels. (Fiddly, but quite possible!) Now you can retrieve the back of the cab and oversew it in place. Next, tackle the front cab pieces (with windows). These need only be stitched where it shows! Part of the one facing forward will be hidden by the boiler and, if you are lining your train, the one facing backwards need only be covered as far as the lining — otherwise stitch it completely. Oversew the forward facing piece to the boiler. Oversew the two pieces together and oversew round the windows. Add the (optional) lining.

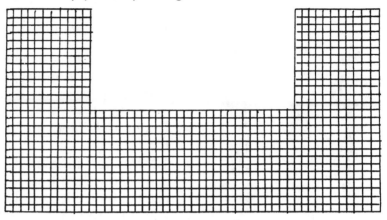

Boiler

Now stand back and admire your handiwork. My guess is that your child will be as delighted as you are!

Note
I have made a smaller version of this train for 'frail' children. This time I used finer, 10 mesh, plastic canvas, single strands of double knitting wool, piping cord size 1 and sausage-shaped buttons instead of toggles. Adjustments were made to the dimensions above to keep the proportions correct.

Button Up a Mobile

Long-lasting

This mobile is a three-in-one toy which, unlike most mobiles, is intended to be hung within reach of the children. Once it is assembled, they can rearrange the pieces as they choose, or just ring the bells and twist it to make it 'mobile'. It combines shape and colour recognition with button training—and looks decorative into the bargain. When in pieces, few children can resist the urge to put it together! It consists of a triangular hanger with sets of three pieces suspended from each corner to make a 'dangle'. Each dangle is finished off with a bell. The various components are attached to each other by means of toggles and loops. The pieces can be sorted and hung in two ways— either colours together (as illustrated) or shapes together.

193

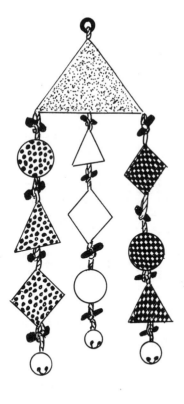

Materials

For the hanger:

- 4 large equilateral triangles in thick card, sides say 15cm (6").
- Fabric for covering them.

For the pieces: Use thin card and cut —

- 6 equilateral triangles, sides say 10 cm (4");
- 6 squares, sides say 8 cm (3");
- 6 circles, diameter say 9 cm ($3\frac{1}{2}$").
- Bright red, blue and yellow fabric for covering them.
- 12 wooden toggles. Some have a groove in the centre, others a hole. Either is suitable but, if you use the type with a hole, make sure the piping cord will go through it.
- 4 m piping cord, say size 3 or 4. This is a generous amount.
- White thread.
- A hanging ring (optional — you can also hang the mobile by a loop).
- 3 large bells.
- Strong adhesive — e.g. U-Hu.

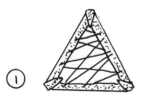

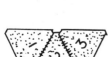

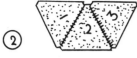

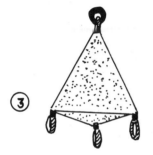

Method

The hanger. Take the four thick card triangles. Snip off the tip of each point. (At the assembly stage this will make a small gap to accommodate the piping cord.) Cover each triangle with fabric, patchwork fashion — stick or stitch. Neaten the points by folding in and pulling the overhanging fabric towards the centre of the triangle. Stick it down (Figure 1). Join three triangles together by oversewing the edges (Figure 2). Fold the triangles into the shape of a tetrahedron to see how the finished hanger will look.

Now make the loops. Cut four lengths of piping cord, about 15 cm (6"). Take one length, thread it through the hanging ring and knot the ends together. Return to the tetrahedron, open it out a little. Put plenty of glue on the knot and close the tetrahedron round it. (The reason for snipping off the ends of the triangles will now be apparent.) The glue on the knot will hold the tetrahedron in shape temporarily while you sew triangle one to triangle three. Next make the other loops. Knot the cord ends together, and make sure each loop is large enough to accept a toggle comfortably. Glue the loops in position. Close up the whole figure by oversewing triangle four to the others (Figure 3).

Next make the 'dangles'. Take two similar shapes of thin card, say circles, to make the back and front of a piece. Cover one side of each with red fabric, patchwork fashion. (Stick or stitch.) Cut lengths of piping cord as before (say 15 cm). You will need 21 in all — two each for the nine pieces and three for the final bells. Take a length and wind it over a toggle. Stitch and bind the cord to hold the toggle firmly in place. Leave about 2 cm ($\frac{3}{4}$") free for sticking inside the piece. Unravel the unbound part of the cord (Figure 4), so that it will lie as flat as possible, and stick it to the inside of one coloured circle. Make a plain loop the same way, by stitching and binding. (Check it is the right size to take a toggle.) Unravel the ends and stick it opposite the toggle (Figure 5). Place the second covered circle over the first and oversew them together, making a few extra stitches for added strength when you come to the piping cord (Figure 6). Repeat the process with all the other pieces, working out the sequence so that you end up with a circle, triangle and square in each colour. Lastly, attach the bells to the remaining toggles. Either use unravelled piping cord or make a buttonhole loop.

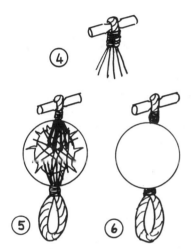

Bows

Tying Shoelaces

Here is a helpful tip for teaching a child to tie a bow. Practise on a real pair of shoes. Acquire two pairs of shoelaces in contrasting colours — e.g. black and white. Tie one black and one white shoelace together, and use this extra long strip to lace up one shoe. (A black end will come out of one top eyelet and white out of the other.) Lace up the other shoe in the same way. Put one shoe in front of your child and the other in front of that — as though they were treading on a line. Put your arms around your child, so that you can reach the front shoe. *Slowly* tie a bow, and let him copy each action as you make it, on the back shoe. Using different coloured laces makes it clear which one passes in front of or through the loop of the other. I learnt this useful trick from an Educational Psychologist, who assured me it was well known — if not to me! She used football laces threaded in a substantial pair of plywood shoe shapes. These were flat, and easy to carry around to different groups of children.

Poppers

Popper Dollies

Long-lasting
R.L.

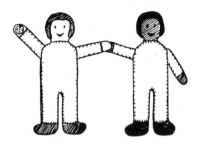

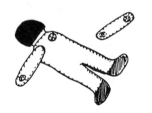

These little people are designed to give a child plenty of practice in pressing together the two parts of a press stud, or 'popper'. They are made from two layers of felt, stiffened with heavy duty iron-on Vilene. Their arms are attached to their bodies with press studs, and there is half another stud sewn to the back of one hand, with the opposite half stitched to the front of the other. With this arrangement, the little people can hold hands and be linked together in a friendly circle (or row).

The colours chosen represent the colours of the rainbow, (red, orange, yellow, green, blue, purple,) plus black and white. The dolls can have their arms arranged in different positions, or even interchanged, so that the yellow doll has red sleeves. If you have the stomach for it, remove all the arms, and jumble them up. Now the children can match up the colours, and return them to their rightful owners, getting plenty of practise in 'popping' on the way.

A Special Noah's Ark
(Illustrated on the cover)

Long-lasting

This toy should only be attempted by people who love sewing! It is very time-consuming — and addictive! The more animals you make, the more you realise you have left out. Each animal is made in profile, with just two legs. Join him, with a press stud, to his mate, and the pair will stand together on their collective four legs. There is some artistic licence here! It would be even more time-consuming to make each animal in its entirety. The children find no problem with the two legged creatures, which can easily be recognised for what they represent. As an educational toy, it has great possibilities. Firstly, the story of the great flood must be told. Then the animals must be paired before they can march into the Ark (plenty of 'popper' practise here), and gradually the children learn the names of all the creatures.

I began with a visit to the Public Library. Here I found plenty of authentic sideways-on pictures of animals, which I could copy for the general outline, and simplify. I aimed to make the animals roughly in proportion but, for practical reasons, the large ones were slightly reduced and the small ones enlarged a little.

A card template of the animal was cut out and used to trace the shape on the heavy duty tack-in Vilene and the felt. (I reversed the template for the second shape so that the pencil marks would be on the inside when the animal was sewn together.) The inside shape was backed with the Vilene and cut out on the line. The outside half was made slightly larger so that, later on, a little stuffing could be inserted to give the animal a slightly rounded and more realistic appearance. One half of a press stud was stitched through the felt and Vilene of the inside half. Any stitching detail, such as the curve of a haunch, wrinkles in the neck, etc., were added to both sides while the shapes were still flat.

Next the two half animals were joined together and the padding worked in. Animals with long legs — or necks! — needed a pipe-cleaner (with its wire ends turned in) to give them extra strength. The second animal was made in the same way but, of course, the press stud was on the opposite side. I found it easier to add eyes and ears when I had a recognisable animal shape to work on, rather than at the flat stage.

The Ark

The collection of pop-together animals need a home. The Ark, which appears on the cover, was made from 7 mesh plastic canvas covered with half cross-stitch worked in two thicknesses of double knitting wool. There are many other ways of making an Ark — from building a card superstructure on a shoebox to using plastic foam covered with fabric. I feel you would not be attempting this toy unless you were familiar with needle and thread, so, with regard to the Ark, I leave you to work out your own solution . . . which may be much better than anything I can suggest!

To add to the potential for imaginative play, the animals should be cared for by Mr and Mrs Noah (and perhaps Ham, Shem and Japhet and their wives?). There are many ways of making the people — from turning them in wood to stitching them in fabric. I made mine by enlarging the finger puppets with arms on p. 82. I extended the bodies and arms by adding a few rows and stitches and used fairly subdued colours to represent natural dyes. I added pipe-cleaners to the arms, so that they could be bent, and stuffed the bodies, but left a space at the bottom for a small plug of dowel. I found this weighted the base of the body and made it stand up properly. I covered the bottom of the dowel plug with a small circle of cloth and stitched it to the hem of the body. Mr Noah was identified by his shepherd's crook (a pipe-cleaner bound in wool) and his long grey beard. Mrs Noah wore a long striped skirt over her knitted body, and a shawl over her shoulders. She carried a tiny bucket (made from the top of a toothpaste tube) for feeding the animals.

See also
Shake and Make, p. 70.

TOYS USING A VARIETY OF FASTENINGS

Australian Cushion

Quick

Take a tip from the Handbook of the Australian Association of Toy Libraries and make a special cushion covered with all sorts of fastenings. Remove the zip from an old pair of trousers; buttons and buttonholes from the front of a discarded dress; lacing holes from a worn-out canvas shoe; find an old belt with a buckle and sew them all firmly to a washable cushion cover. Put the cushion inside, rest it on the table or the child's knee and all the fastenings will be easy to reach. Children react favourably to this trainer, because it contains a variety of fastenings from *real* clothes. Maybe they will recognise the fancy buttons from the front of Auntie Mary's blouse!

Surprise Pockets

Quick

This is an easily made trainer which can be useful with a group of children who need to practise their fastenings. If several are made, each child can have a strip of pockets to explore, and next session she can try another one. In shape, this trainer is similar to a long envelope which has been divided into several sections, or pockets. The flap of the envelope makes the covering for the tops of the pockets and stops the (motivating!) surprises hidden inside from falling out. To lift the flap and find the surprise, a child must first tackle the fastening — button, zip, popper or Velcro.

The easiest way to make the pockets is to start off with a rectangle of material say 20 × 26 cm (8 × 10$\frac{1}{2}$"). Make a hem all round the edge. Put the material wrong side up on the table. Turn the bottom edge up about 10 cm (4") and machine over the hems at the sides to make the long envelope shape with a flap. Lift up the flap, and divide the bag part of the envelope into three pockets by running two rows of stitches from the folded bottom edge to the hem at the top. Sew half a fastening to the front of each pocket and the corresponding half to the flap. If the pockets are made this simple way, the fastenings must *all* be undone before the flap can be lifted. It is a more time-consuming job to attach a separate flap to each pocket, but if you are used to sewing that will be no problem for you.

I used a set of these pockets to good effect with a small group of slow learners. I had a box full of toys for the surprises — a tiny doll in a matchbox, a little plastic car, a homemade scrapbook, a few marbles, a toy watch to wind up and a doodle bag with a squeaker inside. I tried to add to the surprises each week. The children understood that the toys were not for keeping, but that they were entitled to play with them there and then, and the quicker they mastered the fastenings the longer they would have to play! Each child chose a strip of ready filled pockets, and was eager to discover what was inside. Before the session ended, they all returned their toys to the box and chose another set to replace them. These were put in the pockets and the fastenings happily *done up* again ready for the next session.

A Cuddly Cat

Long-lasting

Marianne Willemsen
van Witsen,
Toymaker,
Holland

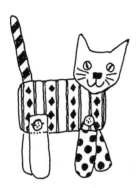

The special feature of this moggie is that its head, legs and tail are all separate pieces which join to the body by means of different fastenings. Marianne says it has a special appeal for the children she calls the 'demolition crew'—the ones who love to take things apart! It also finds favour with the ones who like to put things together and, in the process, they are practising their fastenings.

Materials
- Fabric—strong and washable. Use up odd pieces and don't aim at realism!
- Polyester fibre stuffing.
- Fastenings, e.g. large hook and eye, large press stud, Velcro, buttons.
- Scraps of felt and wool for features.

Method
The body. Cut out a rectangle of fabric approximately 24 × 18 cm ($9\frac{1}{2}$ × 11″). Fold it in half, short sides together. The fold will make the top of the back. Round off the corners. A neat way of doing this is to place a large coin in the corner and draw round it. With right sides together, sew along both sides and part of the way along the tummy, leaving a gap for turning and stuffing. Turn right side out and stuff fairly lightly. Close the gap—oversew or ladder stitch.

The tail. This is like a long finger. Cut the material about 12 × 24 cm (5 × 10″). Fold right sides together, taper the tail at the tip and round it off. Sew it up, turn right side out and stuff.

The head. Copy the picture. As a guide to size, a diagonal measurement from the tip of one ear to the bottom of the chin is approximately 12 cm (5") and the width from cheek to cheek is about 15 cm (6"). Cut out double, for the back and front. Some people find it easier to apply the features at this stage while the material is still flat. With right sides together, sew nearly all the way round, leaving a gap in the chin. Turn right side out, stuff lightly and close the gap. Stitch on the features if you have not already done so.

The legs. Cut these approximately 18 × 12 cm (7 × 5"), but the length may need adjusting according the fastening you use. (Button hole or loop?) Make up the legs in a similar way to the rest of the cat. The picture suggests ways of attaching them.

Finally, sew a Velcro strip to the tail and body (this helps to hold it erect), and attach the head by whatever fastening you choose.

Life-sized Baby Dolls

Long-lasting

Fran Whittle and her team, All Saints Arts and Youth Centre, Sussex

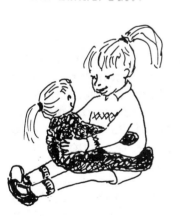

Toys and trainers that help children to manipulate fastenings definitely have their uses, but they are no substitute for the real thing. Fran's dolls can be dressed in proper clothes complete with zips, buttons, poppers and bows, and so help children to practise fastenings in a more lifelike situation.

Materials
- A Babygro, outgrown perhaps, or from the local jumble or car boot sale.
- Stretch fabric for the head. Fran recommends cotton stockinette.
- Polyester stuffing, with the CE safety mark on the pack.
- Wool, felt and thread for hair and features.

Method
First stuff the Babygro. Next make the head. Cut a strip of stretch fabric approximate for the size of the Babygro. (A young baby's body is about $3\frac{1}{2}$ times the length of its head, and its neck is very short.) Stitch the short sides of the stretch fabric together to make

a ring of material. Run a thread along one edge, gather up and fasten off securely. This is the top of the head. Turn the material inside out. Run another thread around the open (neck) end, unthread the needle and leave the thread dangling. Stuff the head, re-thread the needle, draw up the running thread and again fasten off securely. Put the head on top of the Babygro and join them together with several rounds of stitching. The doll will have a floppy head, just like a real baby. This makes it very appealing.

To make the face, first cut the features out of felt. Start with the eyes. These should be half way down the head (or slightly lower) and fairly wide apart. Pin them roughly in place. Do the same with the mouth (and nose?). Then try moving the pieces about a little to see how the expression changes. When you are satisfied, stitch the pieces in place and remove the pins. The hair can be made of wool. One method is to wind it over a piece of stiff paper and machine it down the middle. Cut the wool where it bends round the edges of the paper and tear the paper away. Consider the row of stitching to be the parting, and stitch firmly to the head along this line. Trim off any straggly ends. Select some suitable clothes (with lots of fastenings on them!) from the 'cast offs', and your doll is ready for tender loving care!

Instant Dolls

Loet Vos,
Museum of Childhood,
Toronto

Follow the drawings and within ten minutes you should end up with a rough and ready doll! Just the thing when you want plenty of characters for a model or extra people to live in the dolls' house. Children with good hand function, aged seven and upwards, may be able to make one of these dolls — with a little help in tying the knots. As you see, dressing them is simplicity itself. As an added refinement, pipe-cleaners can be rolled up in the cloth at stage 1 and will add a little stiffening to the arms and legs. Now the arms can be bent and the doll made to sit or kneel. If the arms are made as long as the legs, the doll can be placed on all fours and turned into an animal!

202

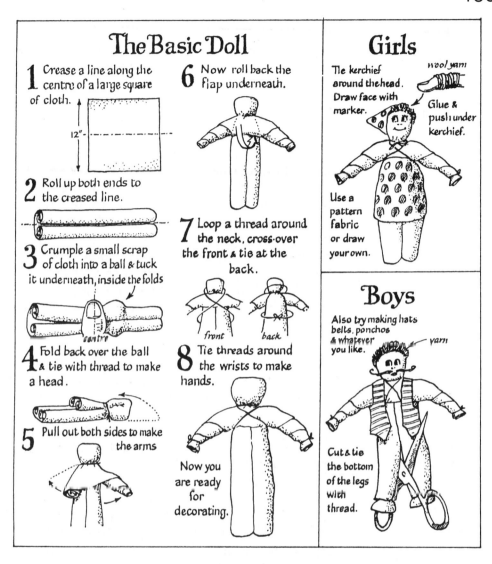

The Basic Doll

1 Crease a line along the centre of a large square of cloth.

12"

2 Roll up both ends to the creased line.

3 Crumple a small scrap of cloth into a ball & tuck it underneath, inside the folds

centre

4 Fold back over the ball & tie with thread to make a head.

5 Pull out both sides to make the arms

6 Now roll back the flap underneath.

7 Loop a thread around the neck, cross-over the front & tie at the back.

front   back

8 Tie threads around the wrists to make hands.

Now you are ready for decorating.

Girls

Tie kerchief around the head. Draw face with marker.

wool yarn

Glue & push under kerchief.

Use a pattern fabric or draw your own.

Boys

Also try making hats belts, ponchos & whatever you like.

yarn

Cut & tie the bottom of the legs with thread.

Sock Dollies

Quick

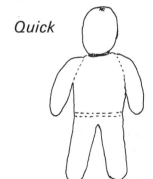

These cuddly little dolls are wonderful as 'extras' for imaginative play. If your child is short of patients for the shoebox hospital beds, here is a quick—and cheap—way to make good the deficit. If you take time to make the clothes removable, you provide yet another opportunity for practice in coping with fastenings.

Cut the foot off a sock and reserve this to make the arms. Think of the rest of the sock as being in three sections—head, body and legs. Pin where you think the neck and hips will be. First make the legs. Lie the sock flat on the table and cut through two thicknesses

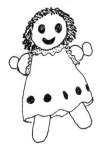

of material, from the ankle end to just below the pins that mark the hips. Round off the tips of the feet. Take out the pins. Turn the sock inside out and stitch up the bottoms of the feet and the inside leg seams. Do this very securely—two rows of stitching—and over-sew the raw edge, otherwise the sock may fray easily and your seams could pull away. Turn the sock right side out. Stuff the legs with polyester fibre, and stitch across the body just above the top of the legs. This helps the dolly to sit down. Stuff the body section and tie (or gather) round the neck. You now have half a doll, with legs and a plump little body, but as yet no head or arms. Run a thread round the top of the sock. Stuff the head and draw up the thread. Fasten off very firmly. Cut two arms from the reserved sock foot. Round off the hand ends and sew them into sausage arms. (Strong seams as before.) Stitch the arms to the body very firmly. Sew on felt features, (or embroider them,) and add wool hair. Cover the head with large French knots for a curly hair style. For a straight cut, wind wool over some thin card, machine or hand stitch down the middle to keep the strands of wool in order. Cut the wool where it bends over the card. Tear the card away from the stitching. Sew the wool hair to the doll, arranging the stitching along the line of the parting.

Make some simple dolls' clothes and play can begin.

The undressed sitting-down doll was made by a nine-year-old. She used the heel of the sock for the doll's sit-upon and cut the legs from part of the foot. She used the rest of the foot to make the arms, and folded down the top of the leg to make the cosy hat.

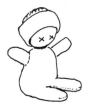

A TOY FOR CHILDREN WITH LIMITED REACH

The Turntable Toy

Long-lasting

The concept of playing on a turntable is not new. For years children with restricted reach have made use of a cake-icing turntable to give them a larger play surface. My turntable, made in wood, has three alternative play 'heads', which provide for plenty of imaginative play combined with fine finger movements. The choice of heads lies between a town layout, a dolls' house and a farm.

Town Layout

The toy began as a town layout for Jenny, a three-year-old with brittle bones. Her movements were very restricted and, because of her small size, she was only able to reach toys about 15 cm away. All her playthings needed to be small and light and, of course, this limited the number of commercial ones on offer. By using a turntable, her play surface was at least doubled, and this opened up exciting possibilities!

The layout was planned on a circle of plywood (diameter approx 30 cm, 12"). A small hill was shaped from an odd scrap of wood and glued to the otherwise flat and rather uninteresting surface. To keep the layout stable, a dowel peg was inserted in the centre of the underside, and this could be located securely in a hole drilled in the turntable. Roadways and grassy areas were painted on the surface of the layout. Houses, shops, a church, school, hospital, etc. were cut from MDF (medium density fibreboard), and a small peg, cut from a cocktail stick, was inserted into the bottom of each. These pegs fitted the small holes drilled at random over the grassy surfaces of the layout. Vehicles, also cut from MDF, included cars, lorries, vans, buses, a milk float, an ambulance, a fire engine, a police car and a removal van—everything the imaginary community could want! These were pegless. They needed to be moved freely along the roadways.

When offered her new toy, Jenny's first reaction was to put the buildings anywhere, often letting them overlap onto the roads in a highly dangerous manner! Then all the vehicles were arranged bumper to bumper in a long, realistic-looking traffic jam. We imagined the feelings of the people stuck in the middle of that! Soon her play became more sophisticated. The buildings were arranged with more thought, and some became the homes of her friends. The school bus did its rounds, visits were exchanged (by car), new neighbours moved in, and the ambulance was constantly required to attend to various catastrophies.

Dolls' House

Next came the dolls' house. This was made open plan for easy access and, by rotating the turntable, Jenny

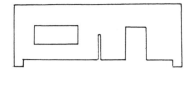

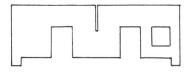

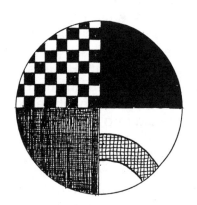

could comfortably reach all parts. Two cross pieces slotted together to make three rooms and a garden area. Doors and windows were cut appropriately and narrow strips removed from the bottoms of the walls, leaving tabs at the ends which fitted the turntable and kept the dolls' house securely in place. The circular floor (also cut from ply) was divided into four segments. A luxurious blue velvet carpet covered the sitting room floor. The kitchen was tiled, and the third room had wall-to-wall hessian for a hard wearing surface. The grass in the garden was green felt and the path cut from a scrap of convincing-looking gravel-coloured vinyl. People were made from pipe-cleaners, heads and hands fashioned from small balls of polyester fibre covered with material from tights and bound on tightly with wool. Scraps of felt, ribbon and lace came in handy for the clothes. Furniture could have been bought, but it was more fun to make our own, Jenny acting in an advisory capacity and doing her bit with felt pens and glue. Matchboxes came in handy for fireplaces and bookshelves. Stamps made splendid pictures, and plastic canvas (from craft shops) covered with wool stitches could convert into almost anything—even an electric stove with an oven door that opened, and a chest with tiny drawers to pull out. Furniture made this way was strong, light and washable.

Given time and a little effort, the dolls' house can develop into a real treasure. As far as imaginative play is concerned, it is the little extras that provide the

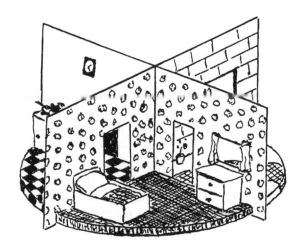

magic. Perhaps the doll child needs a toy box filled with tiny playthings (from crackers?). An apron hanging on the wall would be handy for the doll Mum when she prepares the dinner. Bedding can be made in a jiffy from coloured tissues and, if a wheelchair would add a touch of realism to the play, why not add one from a Playpeople hospital or ambulance set? An exotic rug can be made from a scrap of material with the edges frayed out and, if you are searching for a touch of elegance, why not provide a pot plant made from the cap of a toothpaste tube filled with Polyfilla, and poke in a few minuscule artificial flowers? I am sure I have written enough to start you thinking!

The Farm

The farm was based on the two toys above. Its foundation was a circle of calico, made to fit the top of the turntable. A wide strip of calico sewn to the edge made a straight skirt which held the calico top safely on the turntable. The bottom of the skirt was turned up and stitched vertically here and there to form little pockets. These were handy for storing animals, etc. The circle was divided into four segments (like the dolls' house floor). Several matching segments were made from odd pieces of material in suitable colours and textures, and represented the fields throughout the seasons. (Brown corduroy for a ploughed field, green terry towelling for a grassy meadow, etc.) The fields could be fixed to the calico top with Velcro, and changed as the year progressed. The farm house and outbuildings were made from plastic canvas. The animals were bought plastic ones, and the plywood trees slotted together like the walls of the dolls' house. The hedges were made from strips of foam plastic daubed with acrylic paint. The farm machinery was manufactured, but the sacks of animal feed, bundles of hay, etc. were all homemade and, of course, toothpaste caps came in handy as buckets and an odd scrap of card could soon be fashioned into a feeding trough!

I suppose every toymaker has one favourite creation and the turntable toy—with its developments—is certainly mine. It was fun to make, looked good, and best of all was just right for the child for whom it was first intended. As a bonus, it was equally attractive to all her able-bodied friends who swarmed round it like the proverbial bees round the honey pot! Now Jenny has outgrown it, but it continues to delight other children with limited reach.

TACTILE GAMES

Tactile Ring Game

Long-lasting

This game was invented as a 'trainer' for the party game of 'Pass the Parcel'. A series of large fabric sausages, each with a different filling inside, were joined together with a length of piping cord between each, to form a ring. The children sat in a circle round the ring, and fiddled with the sausage in front of them. When the music started, the sausages were passed from child to child until the music stopped. Pause for another fiddle with a different sausage until the music began again, and the sausages were once more passed from hand to hand. As a co-operation game for very young children, and those with learning difficulties, this one is a winner. The ring of sausages makes a good focus of attention and the different 'feels' (or noisemakers if you prefer) inside each as they rotate round the circle hold the children's interest.

Materials
- Different fabrics for the sausages. Strong, brightly coloured, perhaps textured, but not too thick or the contents cannot be felt. Size approx. 30 cm (12") square.
- Lengths of piping cord for linking the sausages together. Approx. 36 cm (14") long.
- Contents for the sausages, *see* list on p. 149 for inspiration.

Method
Decide on the number of sausages that you need, possibly six to eight. The number of children in the group you have in mind will be the deciding factor. You need one sausage per child and perhaps a couple of spare ones. Cut out the required number of squares

of fabric and corresponding lengths of piping cord. Turn in the ends of each sausage and hold down with a gathering thread. Stitch the sides of the sausage together. (Two rows of stitching advised, for strength.) Tie a *large* knot at each end of a length of piping cord. Put one knot inside the sausage. Gather up the end and use the thread to stitch the cord (just above the knot) firmly in place. Insert contents into the sausage. Gather up as before and stitch firmly. You now have a tactile sausage with piping cord protruding from each end. Repeat the process with another sausage, and add it to a cord from the first one. Continue in this way until the ring is complete. Now all you need is a circle of children to appreciate your efforts!

Tabletop games

Mary was a little girl of six who had recently lost her sight. As her home tutor, it was up to me to help her through the difficult period of adjustment. I needed to make, and sometimes invent, a variety of tactile games which would help her to 'think' through her fingertips. When the time came for her to learn Braille, sensitive fingertips would be essential. We began with adaptations of traditional dominoes and lotto games described in the chapter on 'Making the Most of Sight'.

Tactile Dominoes

Quick

In this game, textures (from the list on p. 151) replaced the normal dots. Tactile dominoes are available commercially, but the tactile areas — presumably for reasons of cost — are always on the small side. This is fine for children who are already used to gaining information through their fingertips, but younger children and those, like Mary, who have been in the habit of using their eyes rather than their fingers, need a larger area to feel. Make your own set of dominoes and the sky is the limit!

Mary's set of tactile dominoes was made from eight rectangles of thick card, each 10 × 20 cm (4 × 8″). I drew a line down the centre of each and arranged the rectangles in a line. Then the fun began! The left hand half of the first rectangle was left blank. Adhesive was smeared, right up to the edges, on the right-hand half, and on the left-hand half of the second rectangle. Both these sticky sections were covered with velvet. The process was repeated with the right and left halves of the second and third rectangles, — this time using sandpaper — and so on all along the line, finishing with a blank.

In play, we would each have four rectangles. In turn, one of us would start the game by putting a rectangle on the table. The other player would hope to find a matching texture among her collection. If no luck, a turn was missed. Ultimately, all the textures would be needed. The sequence of textures was always the same, but it could begin and end in a different place which added a little variety to the game.

Button Dominoes

Long-lasting

Here buttons of distinctive shapes were substituted for textures. They were sewn to rectangles of double felt, and made a more difficult game than the one above.

Materials
- Felt.
- Iron-on Vilene for stiffening.
- Button thread for attaching the buttons firmly.
- As many different pairs of buttons as is suitable for the child in question. For young children use large buttons with very distinctive shapes, and not too many pairs. At a later stage the game can, of course, be made more challenging by introducing more pairs and smaller buttons.

Method
Back the felt with iron-on Vilene. Cut out twice the number of rectangles required for your game. Suggested size of 10 × 5 cm (4 × 2″). Half will hold the buttons, the rest will back them, adding extra stiffness, and covering the stitches which attach the buttons. Arrange the buttons in the usual domino sequence — right-hand side on one rectangle corresponding to the left-hand side of the next. Stitch the buttons on firmly. Add the backing pieces, stick and stitch.

Note

These dominoes will hand wash, but don't put them in with the clothes in case the colour runs.

Another set of these button dominoes was made for three children with a severe visual impairment, but we had a problem. As they played together, it was almost impossible for them to keep the dominoes in line. The solution was easy, thanks to our good friend Velcro! A strip, long enough to hold the line of dominoes was stuck and stitched to felt. This was mounted on a strip of stiff cardboard to give it stability. The other half of the Velcro was cut to size, and sewn to the backing pieces before they were stuck and stitched to the button layer.

Real Things Dominoes

Long lasting

A school for severely visually impaired children near to me needed new toys to add to their toy library.

I remembered a set of Real Things Dominoes designed by Roger Limbrick. The items on his dominoes included hinges, buttons, keys, nylon scouring pads, corks, doorknobs, pencils, metal letters, sliding bolts, bell push buttons, keyhole plates, detergent bottle tops, etc. This list is sufficient to give you the idea.

Materials
- Plywood or medium density fibreboard, say 12 mm.
- Pairs of objects to attach as suggested by the list above, and added to by you. I also included fluffy woolly balls, cotton reels and little toy cars — with their wheels removed so that they would lie flat.
- Very strong adhesive such as Araldite.
- Small screws to use as appropriate.
- Polyurethane varnish to protect the wooden parts.

Method
Cut out and sandpaper the required number of rectangles, say 15 × 7 cm (6 × 3"). Lay out the dominoes in a row and arrange the 'real things' in the best order. Glue (and screw?) them in place. Cover the exposed parts of the wood with polyurethane varnish. As an extra refinement, a strip of Velcro can be stuck to both ends of the dominoes so that, in play, they can be coupled together and cannot be joggled out of line.

Feely Bingo

Quick

This game is similar to ordinary Bingo, or Lotto, but (yes, you've guessed it!) textures replace the number or pictures. To make a game for three, you will need six fairly large sheets of stiff card, three for the master cards and three to cut up. Raid your rag bag for scraps of suitable material and consult the list on p. 151. Take a master card and stick on about four squares of contrasting textures — say sandpaper, fur fabric, velvet and lino tile. Repeat these textures on another card, and cut this one into four pieces, so that each can be matched to the ones on the master card. Repeat the process with the other cards, using different textures on each pair.

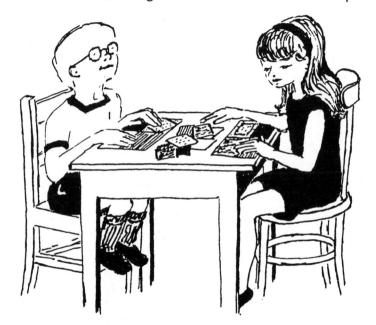

To play, all the small cards are placed face downwards in the middle of the table. Each player has a master card and takes it in turns to pick a small one from the centre. If it matches a texture on his card, he keeps it and puts it on the appropriate place. If it does not match, he returns it to the centre — and so on until all the cards are full.

Note
If a small card is lost the game is useless, so it is worthwhile, at the making stage, to provide a box or bag for all the pieces.

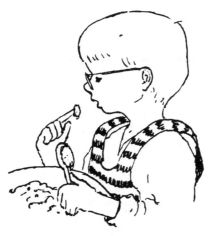

Making the most of TASTE

IT IS IMPOSSIBLE TO ENTER A SHOP AND FIND a tasty toy! This does not mean that the sense of taste should be overlooked as a possible source of fun. It is up to us to fill the gap.

The following pages suggest ways of making the most of taste. There are ideas for using food in unusual ways. The recipes — for safety reasons — require no heating or the use of electrical mixers. Most children who can use both hands can attempt them all. Even those with a hand-function problem may be able to mash a banana with a fork if the basin is supported on a Dycem mat. Glance through, and see what might be possible for the child in question. The cooking will be fun, and the end product is sure to be tasty!

FUN WITH FOOD

Apple Boats

One apple makes two boats. Wash the apple and cut it in half. Scoop out the core with a spoon. Cut a square of paper to be a sail. Fix it to the boat with a cocktail stick.

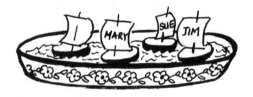

For a party, arrange the boats on a bed of chopped-up lime jelly to represent the sea, and write a child's name on each sail.

Cheese and Pineapple Hedgehogs

You will need:

- A good sized potato (makes two hedgehogs).
- Cheddar cheese.
- A small tin of pineapple chunks.
- Cocktail sticks.
- Baking foil.

Cut the potato in half and wrap both pieces in baking foil. Cut the cheese into small cubes. Drain the pineapple chunks and drink the juice! Thread cubes of cheese and pineapple chunks alternately onto the cocktail sticks. (Say three on each.) Push them into the foil-covered potatoes to represent the spines on the hedgehog's back. Raisins can be used to make its eyes. Fix them in with little pieces of cocktail stick.

Growing a Cress Hedgehog

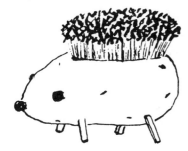

You will need:

- A fairly large potato — roughly hedgehog-shaped.
- 4 dead matchsticks.
- A little cotton wool.
- Some cress seeds.

Using a teaspoon, scoop out a hollow in the middle of the potato, where the prickles should grow. Snip the burnt heads off the matches. Poke two into the front of the potato to make the eyes, and one at the very front to be the nose. Poke the headless matchsticks into the bottom to be the legs. Fill the scooped-out top with cotton wool, and dampen this well. Sprinkle fairly liberally with cress seeds. Stand the hedgehog in a light, warm place, where he can be admired. Water him daily, and soon he should have a splendid crop of cress prickles growing on his back. This can be harvested, washed and eaten with ceremony.

A Hairy Humpty Dumpty

This is a variation of the Cress Hedgehog. Start with an empty egg shell left over from the breakfast boiled egg. Wash it and sit it in an egg cup so that it is easier to handle. Stuff it with moist cotton wool.

215

Give it a cheerful face (felt pens) and sprinkle on the seeds. Make sure the cotton wool never dries out, and before long Humpty should have a spectacular hair-do!

Fabergé Eggs

Pam Rigley,
Teacher and toymaker

Perhaps you have marvelled at these bejewelled creations, designed to give pleasure to the rich and famous. Children can decorate eggs too. Made as presents, they will probably give just as much pleasure to the less rich and famous!

First blow the egg by making a hole in each end with a pin and enlarging one hole slightly by waggling a pin around inside it. This will also prick the membrane of the yolk. Hold the egg over a basin and blow through the small hole to eject the contents. Wash out the egg shell as thoroughly as possible. Cover the small hole with Sellotape. Fill the egg shell, a little at a time, with a fairly sloppy mixture of Polyfilla. When this has set, the egg can be safely handled by a child.

Now for the decoration. Perhaps a face suggests itself. Felt pens to the fore. Then extra refinements can be added — like a fur fabric top knot, bead earings or a felt collar. An older child with agile fingers may want to cover her egg with an elaborate design instead of a face. She might use 'spaghetti' ribbon — the very narrow woven one — to divide the shell into sections and fill these with patterns of sequins and tiny beads.

Note
PVA adhesive is suitable for a quick fix, but after a while the decorations tend to fall off. Use a stronger adhesive like U-Hu.

Making Butter

You will need:

- A glass or plastic jar with a well-fitting top and a wide neck. The container must be transparent, so the children can see the butter forming. A plastic squash bottle *can* be used, but it is difficult to extract the butter through the narrow neck.
- The cream from the top of the milk.
- A pinch of salt.
- A knife.
- Plain biscuits on which to spread the butter.

Making butter can be a tedious process, but it is fun if several children take turns with the shaking. If a glass jar is involved, supervision is necessary.

Put the top of the milk and the pinch of salt in the jar and fix the lid on properly. The children can sit in a circle, taking it in turns to shake the jar. Perhaps this can be done to singing, like the work songs and sea shanties of the past, the jar being shaken in time to the rhythm like maracas! At first the milk becomes bubbly, but gradually little blobs of cream collect together on the surface when the shaking stops. Finally, these form one big lump. Spread this on the biscuits and have a feast.

Pasta

Pasta comes in a great variety of shapes — twirls, bows, shells, catherine wheels, quills and so on. These can be mounted on card or the (well washed) polystyrene trays used to package meat and vegetables. PVA adhesive will stick the pasta to them efficiently. Colour can be added to the pasta with food colouring. Put a few drops in a little water, soak the pasta in it for only a few minutes, then spread it out to dry. When all the water has evaporated, and it is firm again, it is ready for use.

Teddy Bear's Picnic

I remember one very wet afternoon when our family morale was definitely in need of an uplift. We decided it was Big Ted's birthday. Every doll and stuffed animal

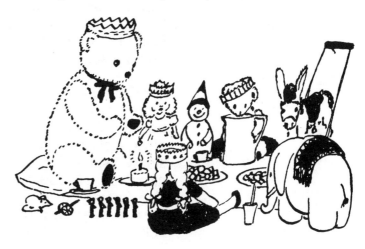

in the house was collected and arranged on cushions around a tablecloth spread on the floor. The big ones propped up the little ones and all were dressed in their party best. Paper crowns were made from strips of coloured paper cut with pinking shears and decorated with gummed paper shapes or felt pens. Table napkins were made from paper tissues. The party guests obligingly listened to tapes while the feast was prepared by the children. All the food was miniature. Little star biscuits, tiny Marmite sandwiches, miniature carrot sticks, raisins and peanuts were arranged on the (newly washed!) plates from the dolls' tea set and, of course, all were completely cleared before the party was over.

Incidentally, this can be a wonderful way to coax a convalescent to eat without seeming to make a fuss. One mother I know adds to the fun by putting a few drops of food colouring in the milk which is poured from the toy tea pot.

RECIPES WHICH DO NOT REQUIRE COOKING

Tempting a Reluctant Eater

Parents of 'faddy' children know that serving a meal in an unusual way can sometimes help to make the food more appealing. Involving a child in the preparation of the food can also help. Play has been known to turn mealtimes into something to look forward to instead of that dreaded battle of wills!

Here are some ideas to start you off.

1. *A salad face*
   Watercress makes excellent curly hair. Use hard boiled egg slices for the eyes. If the yoke is not always central you can have saucy eyes looking sideways, looking upwards (seeking inspiration?), cast demurely downwards, or even horrific squints! Use tomato slices to make rosy cheeks, a radish for a coquettish mouth and lettuce or cress for a collar.

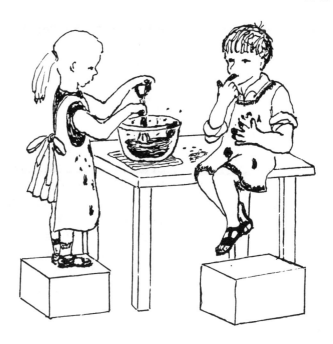

2. *Fruit flowers*
   Apple or orange segments can be arranged in the shape of flowers. Grapes, cut in half and the pips removed, make good centres.

3. *Shapes cut in cheese*
   Squares of processed cheese are ideal for artistic expression. They are easy to cut with a blunt knife and might suggest a house shape. Cut out the door and windows, and put a pitch on the roof (eating the trimmings of course!), and there you are.

Open Sandwiches

These make a change from ordinary sandwiches, and are popular with visiting children who can see what they are getting! They are unsuitable for children who are not too adept at handling food, as the toppings tend to fall off.

Start with a slice of bread, crispbread, toast or a roll. Spread butter or margarine and add a topping, e.g. cheese, egg, sardine, liver sausage, Marmite. Add lettuce, cress, tomato or watercress to add a little 'crunch'. For a sweet topping, honey and dates or jam and cream cheese were top favourites in this house. My neighbour showed me how to make a few strawberries go a very long way. Cut the buttered bread in strips, cut the strawberries in thin slices and arrange them on the strips. Lightly dust with sugar.

Sandwich Fillings

These can be made 'according to taste', and can be prepared by children. All they have to do is mash everything together with a fork in a deep basin, so that the ingredients combine to make a fairly stiff spread. Quantities have purposely been kept vague. If a child does not like salad cream, leave it out and add a little more tomato. A little butter or margarine or a few drops of milk can always be added to a spread if it is too stiff, but add very sparingly in case the spread suddenly becomes too sloppy or greasy.

1. *Meat Spread*

   Ingredients
   - A small tin of corned beef or meat loaf.
   - A tomato, peeled and chopped, or tomato puree.
   - Salad cream.
   - A pinch of salt and a shake of pepper.

   Chop up the meat so that it will mash more easily. Put it in a basin. Add a *small* amount of chopped tomato (or purée), salad cream, salt and pepper. Mash all the ingredients together with a fork until they are well mixed. Season to taste and gradually add more tomato or salad cream until the concoction is smooth enough to spread.

2. *Cheese and Tomato Spread*

   Ingredients
   - Grated cheese.
   - A teaspoonful of chutney.
   - A tomato.
   - A pinch of salt and a shake of pepper.

   Grate the cheese. (A Multi Mouli Grater is safe for children to use. They cannot hurt their knuckles on the cutting surface which is enclosed in a case.) Put it in a basin, and gradually stir in the chutney and a little skinned and chopped tomato until the mixture is soft enough to spread.

3. *Egg and Cheese Spread*

Ingredients
- Hard boiled egg.
- Some grated cheese.
- Salad cream.
- A pinch of salt and shake of pepper.

Chop up the egg and put it in a basin with the grated cheese. Add a little salad cream and mash them all together with a fork.

Banana Milk Shake

(Makes two big ones)

Ingredients
- 1 banana.
- 2 scoops of ice cream.
- 1 rounded tablespoon sugar (optional).
- 1 pint of milk.

Peel the banana. Put it in a basin and mash it with a fork. Add the milk and sugar. Hand whisk until it is well mixed and frothy. Pour into two glasses and add a scoop of ice cream to each. Drink through a thick straw before the ice cream melts.

Bugs on a Log

This is an American idea for older children with strong teeth! Wash, trim and cut some celery into lengths of about 5 cm (2") to represent the logs. Fill each 'log' with cottage or cream cheese, and make the 'bugs' from raisins or peanuts.

Fresh Fruit Salad

Mix chopped/sliced/grated fruit with unsweetened fruit juice. Young children can grate apple or slice banana with a blunt knife.

Gooseberry Fool

Ingredients
- A tin of gooseberries, or fresh, stewed ones.
- Custard—tinned or freshly made.
- A little caster sugar.

Use a hand whisk to mix all these together until they

are well blended. (Provide a deep basin, or an enthusiastic cook might spray the mixture everywhere.) Pour the mixture into individual glasses and decorate with half a glacé cherry. Chill in the fridge.

Fruit Cream

Ingredients
- $\frac{1}{2}$ lb (225 g) soft fruit — raspberries, black currants, strawberries, etc.
- $\frac{1}{2}$ lb (225 g) plain cottage cheese.
- 2 small cartons natural yoghurt.

Put a large sieve over a deep basin and press all the ingredients through with the back of a spoon. Stir them all together so that they are well mixed. Put in individual glasses and chill.

Fondant Creams

Icing sugar and a *very little* white of egg mixed together make a firm dough which can be moulded into shapes or rolled out and cut with a blunt knife or small metal or plastic cutters. Decorate the sweets with a tiny piece of glacé cherry or an edible silver ball, etc. and lay them out to dry on a sheet of greaseproof paper, which has been sprinkled with icing sugar to stop them from sticking to it. Arrange the sweets in individual paper cases to give to Granny as a present!

Flavour and colour can be added if you wish. Peppermint, lemon juice or coffee essence are the usual choice. (To make coffee essence, mix a small amount of instant coffee with a *very little* boiling water to make a concentrated solution.)

As a Christmas treat, this mixture can be used to make snowmen or old-fashioned sugar mice with long string tails.

Note
An easy way for a child to separate the white of an egg from the yolk is to break the egg on a plate, place an egg cup over the yolk, and slide the white off the plate into a basin.

Stuffed Dates

Remove the stone from each date. Make a small sausage of fondant cream (*see* above) — about the size of the date stone — and pop this inside the date. Top it with a small piece of glacé cherry or walnut.

222

Coconut Ice

Ingredients
- 8 oz (225 g) desiccated coconut.
- 8 oz (225 g) icing sugar.
- A small tin of sweetened condensed milk.
- Food colouring — pink is usual.

Mix the desiccated coconut and icing sugar together. Put half aside. Gradually add about one tablespoon, or less, of sweetened condensed milk to the other half to make a very stiff mixture. Put about the same amount of sweetened condensed milk in a cup. Add the colouring and stir it in well. Add the pink milk to the dry mixture you set aside. Sprinkle a tin with icing sugar and press the mixture into it, keeping the colours separate. Leave it to set while everyone has a good wash! A session with a toothbrush is a good idea too!

Marzipan Sweets

Buy a pack of ready-made marzipan and get busy. Mould the marzipan into tiny fruit shapes. These can be delicately coloured by painting them with diluted food colouring. (Use a clean paint brush!) People can be fashioned and painted, or the marzipan can be cut into shapes with a blunt knife or small pastry cutters. Ornament them with raisins, small pieces of glacé cherry, etc. Sprinkle a sheet of greaseproof paper with icing sugar. Put the marzipan shapes on it to dry.

A Pudding for the Birds

Quick

All you need is a yogurt pot, scraps of bird-favourite food, some melted fat to bind them all together and either some string or some small mesh nylon net (once used to hang up peanuts or to package satsumas, etc.) to hang up the finished pudding. If you use the string method, tie one end to a crust and push it to the bottom of the yogurt pot. Fill the rest of the pot with scraps of fat meat, peanuts, breadcrumbs, etc. Make sure the string is in the middle and coming out of the top of the pot. *You* pour over melted fat to cover all the bits and pieces. Put in a cool place to set. Turn it out of the yogurt pot (if it has set very firmly, you may need to run it under the hot tap for a second), and hang it where it can be watched from the window.

223

SOME GROUP GAMES INVOLVING FOOD
AND THE SENSE OF TASTE

Hocus Pocus

I was taught this game by a Swiss friend who was an Occupational Therapist in a children's hospital. I suspect she invented it. It can be a favourite with all young children who are mature enough to take turns. It has a perfect formula—a ritual sentence, eating sweets, and everyone can be a winner! It is most successful when played with a small group so that turns come round quite quickly. Imagine a little bunch of children gathered round a leader who has on her lap a plate, a teaspoon and a bag of (very!) small sweets. One child is chosen. He runs to the corner of the room and hides his eyes. The leader puts three sweets on the plate, say a red, a green and an orange one. The children gather round the leader chant the ritual sentence 'Hocus Pocus, don't eat *me*'. At *me* the leader points to a sweet, say the red one. That has now become 'magic'. The chosen child comes from the corner and tries to guess which is the magic sweet. If he points to the green or orange ones, he may eat those. If he points to the magic red one, he may eat that one but *no more*! Whatever his choice, he is certain to have one sweet. If he is lucky, he may have two or even three if he picks the magic one last. The watching children become very involved in the game, clapping the lucky guesses, and groaning when

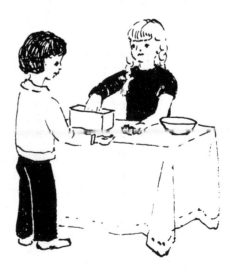

the magic sweet is chosen. At the end of the game, it is time to share out the remainder of the sweets.

The game can be played equally well with small pieces of fruit or different-shaped breakfast cereals.

Shop Treasure Hunt

This game was a 'must' at all our family birthday parties. The 'treasure' (butterbeans, or rice when the children were older) was exchanged for small sweets at the 'shop', but peanuts, crisps or raisins could be used equally well.

The 'treasure' was hidden all over the house. The children searched for it and could exchange it at the 'shop' at the current rate, e.g. one bean = one sweet, or there could be more complicated bartering like three grains of rice for two peanuts or one large crisp. The rules were different every year! Everyone had a turn at being shopkeeper, and the treasure was surreptitiously re-hidden as long as stocks lasted. It was a good idea to issue the stock by degrees. Some shopkeepers when left on their own were inclined to take a quick profit!

Yummy Yum

This is a tasting game popular at parties for older children who can write. All are blindfolded, and each is given a plate containing small pieces of favourite foods. These might include a peanut, a raisin, a slice of apple, banana, cucumber, a tiny biscuit, a crisp, etc. When everyone has finished consuming their ration, they remove their blindfolds and make a list of as many of the tastes as they can remember.

The Chocolate Game

This game is a certain winner for an able-bodied group of older children. If you don't want to play it as described, just make up your own rules!

Before the game begins, you need to collect a die and a tray (to catch the die when thrown), a hat, scarf and pair of gloves, a bread board or a tin pate, a blunt knife and fork, and several small bars of chocolate. (This is more hygienic than using a large one. You will see the sense of this if you read on.)

The children sit in a circle. The bar of chocolate and everything else are on a table in the middle. Someone carries the tray and die to each child in turn. If someone throws a six, it is the signal for that player to rush to the table, put on the hat, scarf and gloves and attack the bar of chocolate with the knife and fork. This is the only permissable way of eating it. Meanwhile, the children in the circle continue to throw the die in turn. As soon as a six comes up, that player rushes to the table. This is the signal for the child already there to stop eating and remove all the clothes, so that the new player can put them on and have a go at the chocolate. Sometimes there is not enough time to put on all the clothes before another six is thrown, so the fun becomes fast and furious.

Replace the chocolate bars as necessary, and keep some in reserve for those who do not manage to eat some during the game.

MAKING THE MOST OF THE KITCHEN

So far, this chapter has been concerned with the sense of taste and having fun with food. Most of the action has taken place in the kitchen. It is worthwhile considering this room, the hub of the household, as a potential play space. It has an easily-cleaned floor, running water, and cuboards full of readymade toys...... sieves to rub with a metal spoon, egg cups to stack, unopened packets of food to build with and lids to fit to saucepans and sturdy baking tins to bang with a wooden spoon. What child could ask for more?

Of course, there are moments such as jam-making days and all other times when scalding hot pans are around, when children must be firmly excluded from the kitchen, or at least confined to a safe area. The kitchen can make the perfect place for adults and children to enjoy each other's company when cooking is not in progress, and low cupboards have had their handles tied together or have been filled with harmless objects (like saucepans and baking tins), and all dangerous items like bleach, knives and glass bottles have been stored well out of reach.

The following descriptions of 'kitchen play' show how children can be amused happily and usefully, while the essential work of running the household continues.

Two-Dimensional Magnetic Toys

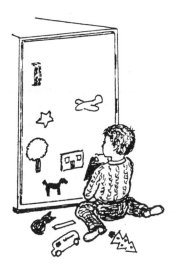

All kitchens have useful metal surfaces like the fridge or a large tin tray. These can be used to make a splendid play surface for magnetic shapes. Once small strips of magnetic tape or undecorated disc fridge magnets have been applied to the backs of thick card or plywood shapes, they will cling to any vertical metal surface in a very satisfactory way. The use of magnetic toys can be particularly helpful for children with hand co-ordination difficulties. The homemade ones suggested below can have just the right amount of magnetism added to make them grip the metal surface easily. If necessary, extra magnetism can be added to give a stronger bond.

If you already have a set of plastic or wooden shapes, use these to make a simple magnetic toy. The shapes can be stuck to the fridge door and shunted around to sort for colour matching or for pattern making. If you are involved with a toy library or play group, the chances are there will be a set of well scribbled-over plywood farm or zoo animal templates, or even a set of vehicle shapes which have seen better days. Give them a new lease of life by painting one side and applying a magnet (tape or disc), to the back — perhaps two if the template is heavy. Increase the play value by adding your own cut-out card shapes of trees, houses, farm buildings, people, street furniture like 'phone and post boxes, or whatever seems appropriate.

Note
Magnetic tape can be obtained from Educational Suppliers (p. 4). It can also be bought from some tool shops, large stationers or firms dealing with advertising and display equipment. Small disc magnets for applying to homemade fridge ornaments can be bought from suppliers of craft materials.

Playing at the Sink

Mrs A. is about to tackle a very grubby wash. The family had a picnic on the common yesterday and all that tree climbing and playing on the grass has left the tee shirts and jeans in a very sorry state. Gareth is a six-year-old who has Down's Syndrome. His school is closed today and he wishes he had his big brothers to play with. Mrs A. decides to make a pie for supper before she tackles the washing, but first she must think of a way to keep Gareth busy and happy. She looks at the pile of dirty washing. Nothing could possibly make it worse, so today is the ideal day for a 'water frolic'. She fetches a low stool and places it in front of the sink. She surrounds this with the dirty washing to mop up the inevitable flood. She half fills the sink with tepid water. Luckily the day is very warm so Gareth can remove his shoes and socks and most of his clothes. Full of anticipation for the delights to come, he consents to wear his mother's plastic apron and climbs on the stool. Mrs A. gives him a colander. He spends several minutes pressing it into the sink and watching the water well up through the holes. Then comes the best bit! He lifts the colander high and watches the water gush out.

Meanwhile Mrs A. assembles the ingredients for her pie. The colander begins to lose its appeal and any moment it may be held over the dirty washing! Mrs A.

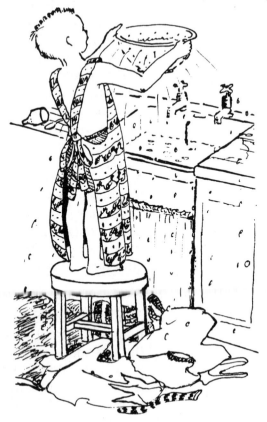

has an instinct for such moves and, before taking away the colander, hands Gareth his favourite water toy. This is a detergent bottle that has been cut in half. The bottom section makes a useful water scoop and the top part, inverted, makes a splendid funnel. Gareth has learnt to put his finger over the stopper hole while he fills the funnel with water from a large spoon. This is a useful exercise for him and he concentrates hard on keeping the spoon level while he spoons the water from the basin into the funnel. Then comes the joyous moment when the funnel is nearly full and he can take his finger away to release the water. He holds it high so that the water will have a long drop. Quite a lot of it runs down his arm and is absorbed by the grubby clothes below. Gareth fills the funnel again. When he tires of this, his mother gives him a handful of corks. He spends some time trying to force these to sink. However often he pokes them to the bottom, as soon as he takes his fingers away they bob to the surface again. Magic!

Mrs A. has finished her pie and has saved the pastry scraps for Gareth to play with later. She is about to throw away the lid of a margerine tub when she has a brainwave. She reaches in a drawer for a paper bag and a cocktail stick. She tears a tiny paper sail, threads it on the cocktail stick which acts as a mast and attaches it to the lid with a blob of pastry. She shows Gareth how to blow gently and make the little raft sail across the sink. He finds this difficult, but is pleased when he achieves modest success. Suddenly, he tires of water play and snatches at the plug. He chuckles as the little raft swirls madly round the plug hole. Mrs A. now tackles the washing while Gareth turns his attention to the pastry scraps.

Just Being Companionable

Mrs B. has Mary home for the weekend. Mr B. has taken lively little Peter to 'help' with the shopping, and later on other members of the family will be coming to tea. Mary lies on her mattress in the corner of the kitchen, out of the draught. She has very limited movement and her sight is poor. At teatime, she will sit in her special chair so that she can be included in the party. Today her mother has moved the breakfast

229

stools into the hall and pushed the table to one side so that Mary can watch her cook. Mary is lying on her left side so that her 'good' arm is free to move. Every time Mrs B. passes by, she shakes her hand and Mary smiles. Before Mrs B. starts to mix a cake, she fixes a piece of string across Mary's corner and hangs up a new rattle. It is like a plastic hand mirror with a reflective surface on one side and a few seeds between the front and back. These make a pleasant, soft sound when shaken. Mary clenches her fist and punches the rattle, making it swing on its string. She appreciates the noise and the reflected light from the mirror surface. When the cake is ready for the oven, Mrs B. starts to clear away the paraphanalia. She is about to wash out the mixing bowl when she remembers Mary. She tucks a tea towel under her chin, rolls up her left sleeve and props the basin at a convenient angle. Then she guides Mary's fist round the bowl to help her suck off the delicious cake mixture. The smell of the baking cake fills the kitchen as Mrs B. starts to clean Mary and the mixing bowl.

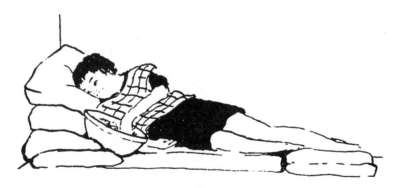

NURSERY RHYMES AND JINGLES WITH FOOD AS THEIR THEME

Pat-a-Cake

Pat-a-cake, pat-a-cake, Baker's man,
Bake me a cake as fast as you can.
Pat it and prick it and mark it with B,
And put it in the oven for Baby and me.

Mix the Pancake

Mix the pancake,
Stir the pancake,

Pop it in the pan.
Fry the pancake,
Toss the pancake,
Catch it if you can!
(Make the appropriate actions.)

**Chop, Chop,
Chippity-Chop**

Chop, chop, chippity-chop,
Cut off the bottom,
And cut off the top.
What there is left we will
Put in the pot:
Chop, chop, chippity-chop.
(The vegetables are being cut up to the make the soup,
in time to the words, make chopping movements with
the side of the hand.)

**Slice, Slice, the
Bread Looks Nice**

Slice, slice, the bread looks nice.
Spread, spread butter on the bread.
On the top put jam so sweet
Now it's nice for us to eat.

**Five Currant Buns
in a Baker's Shop**

Five currant buns in a baker's shop,
Round and fat with sugar on the top,
Along came a boy with a penny one day,
Bought a currant bun and took it away.

Four currant buns .... etc
(Illustrate this with fingers, or let five children represent
the buns.)

**Five Little Peas in
a Pea Pod Pressed**

Five little peas in a pea pod pressed,
(Clench the fingers on one hand.)
One grew, two grew, and so did all the rest.
(Raise fingers to fit the words.)
They grew and grew and did not stop
(Stretch all the fingers wide.)
Till all of a sudden the pod went POP!
(Give a loud clap on the final word.)

Five Little Lollipops

Five little lollipops
Fixed upon a stick,
Shall we have a taste of one?
Lick, lick, lick.

Four little lollipops
Fixed upon a stick ..... etc

Rosy Apples

Five rosy apples by the cottage door,
One tumbled off a twig, and then there were four.

Four rosy apples hanging on a tree,
The farmer's wife took one, and then there were three.

Three rosy apples, what shall I do?
I think I'll have one, and then there'll be two.

Two rosy apples hanging in the sun,
You have the big one, and that will leave one.

One rosy apple, soon it is gone:
The wind blew it off the branch, and now there is none!

Fat Sausages

Five fat sausages sizzling in the pan,
One went 'pop' and the other went BANG!

Four fat sausages sizzling in the pan .... etc

Betty Botter Bought Some Butter

Betty Botter bought some butter. 'But', she said, 'this butter's bitter. If I put it in my batter, it will make my batter bitter, but if I buy better butter, it will make my batter better!'

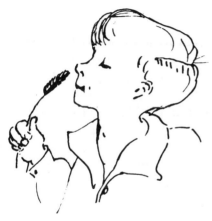

Making the most of SMELL

THE SENSE OF SMELL IS PERHAPS THE LEAST *obviously* stimulating and useful of all the five senses, but it can give much pleasure and, for children with a visual impairment, it can also be extremely useful as a mobility aid. Imagine you know these two children. Michael is seven and has multiple disabilities. If a few drops of perfume are sprinkled on his pillow, he will make a big effort to turn his head to enjoy the smell. Mark is ten and attends a school for the visually impaired. During the holidays he often shops with his mother. He has never been known to confuse the butcher's shop with the baker's for he can confidently distinguish them by smell. He has learnt to trust his nose to confirm much of the information he receives through his ears and fingers. Between these two children, with their special problems, there lies a huge group of others, each with their own personal difficulties. For all of them their lives can be enriched if they make the most of every sense — and that means including the sense of smell.

LEARNING TO SMELL

We notice when a baby has learnt to focus, because we see her stare at something interesting, or look into our eyes and smile back at us. We know she is aware of sounds when she turns her head to investigate a sound behind her. Her delight in her sense of touch is obvious when she starts to grasp, poke and stroke all the interesting textures she finds and, of course, at mealtimes she makes it crystal clear that some tastes please her more than others. The development of her sense of smell is less obvious. If you offer her a flower and invite her to enjoy its perfume, she will probably wrinkle up her nose, but instead of sniffing will snort or snuffle! Perhaps she just lacks control over her breathing. By the time she has become fully mobile and increasingly skilful with her hands, she may discover that ecstatic experience of unscrewing the lids from her mother's cosmetic jars and we find her sniffing appreciatively at their pleasant perfumes. As she grows older, smells will have certain associations, will help to enrich her memories and perhaps even warn her of danger. Every adult has a mental catalogue of smells which has been built up over the years, and many of these will have been first experienced in childhood. Perhaps the smell of new leather shoes is associated with stiff, shiny sandals on the first day of the summer term, or the smell of mud flats at low tide with a happy holiday. When we think about smells, we realise we all have our own particular likes and dislikes, just as we do with sights, sounds, feels and tastes.

Unless we provide our children with plenty of opportunities to explore and experiment, they will find it difficult to discover what they really like.

HELPING CHILDREN ENJOY THE SENSE OF SMELL

How can children with special needs be helped to develop and enjoy the sense of smell? Parents who hope to solve the problem by visiting a toy shop will find there are scarcely any smelly toys available. Smells are such transitory things, literally carried away on the wind, that any toy manufacturer, no matter how enterprising, would be hard put to it to add a universally acceptable and long-lasting one to his product. This means that those of us concerned with the play needs of the children who need our help must make a conscious effort to introduce some smells into their play—in the same way as we think about providing colour, sound and texture.

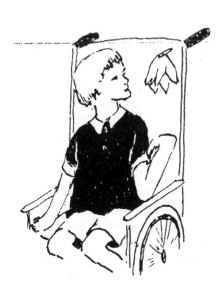

We can make use of activities and games which include different perfumes—some well-tried ones are described in this chapter—but perhaps the richest source of stimulating smells is the child's own environment. One imaginative teacher takes her non-ambulant children to lie in the long grass at the end of the school garden. Imagine the delight of being surrounded by tall waving grasses and to smell the warm earth and the hay—surely a pleasant change from disinfectant and soap suds! In the winter, the same teacher would buy a packet of dried herbs from the supermarket, put some in a little bag made from thin material, and hang it near a child. Without this forethought, the child may never have had the chance to smell mint or bay leaves or basil. A parent who uses our toy library borrowed the pastry kit and made some play pastry for her child. To begin with he was not at all interested, but then she remembered his passion for the smell of peppermint and added a few drops to the dough. That triggered his interest, and he began happily playing with his special pastry, squeezing, prodding and rolling it, and finally chopping it into little pieces with a plastic paper knife.

It takes imagination and an empathy with the child to think of such ways of stimulating the sense of smell. Even the everyday experience of going shopping can be made into an exciting outing of aromatic discovery! Imagine you can watch the mothers in the two following situations and draw your own conclusions!

Mrs A. is going shopping with Peter who is four years old and has very little sight. She is in a hurry today, because her friend is coming to tea, and she has had a frustrating morning. The shops are not far away, but to save time she pops Peter in the buggy and walks there as quickly as possible, hurrying over her selection of food at the supermarket and remembering to buy the bottle of white spirit for her husband. On the way home, her plastic bag is in danger of splitting with the weight of all her purchases, so she gives the white spirit and a bottle of lemonade to Peter to hold, one in each arm, as he sits in the buggy. When she reaches home, she takes them from him and Peter hears her put them on the kitchen table with the other shopping. She turns her attention to helping Peter with his coat and gloves, answers the 'phone and puts the buggy away. The door bell rings. It is the milkman calling for his money. Meanwhile, Peter fancies a drink of lemonade. He knows the bottle is on the table. He remembers it is tall and heavy, because he nursed it all the way home. Confidently, he reaches on the shelf for his mug and places it on the draining board. He takes the nearest bottle, unscrews the lid and begins to pour. Luckily, Mrs A. returns to the kitchen at that moment — so disaster is averted!

Mrs B. is also going shopping, taking with her the baby and four-year-old Lucy who is without sight. Her shopping list is not long today; just white spirit, lemonade, toilet soap, fish and some parsley for the sauce. Lucy walks briskly along, holding on to the handle of the pram. She knows when she is nearly at the end of her road, because the man who lives in the last house has planted an evergreen hedge. This has a special smell and tickles her fingers as she drags them through the young bushes. The man is busy

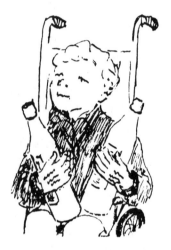

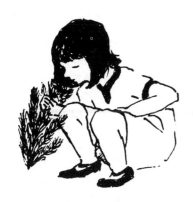

gardening. She can hear his shears cutting the grass border on the other side of the hedge. He calls a greeting and the shopping expedition is diverted through the front gate. He wants to show Lucy how well his herb garden is growing, so they all troop round to the side of the house. Here Lucy, (who can already identify sage, parsley and mint) is delighted to examine a little bush of rosemary, crushing a few leaves between her fingers to increase the smell. They go on their way, Mrs B. with a bag of parsley for the sauce, and Lucy with a little posy of herbs to plant in a saucer garden when she reaches home.

Further down the street, they pause to make way for the delivery man who is carrying a large tray of freshly-baked rolls into the baker's shop. They smell so good that Mrs B. and Lucy decide to buy some. Later, in the supermarket, Lucy helps to push the trolley to the corner where the coffee grinder is kept. Mrs B. selects the beans she wants, takes one out and gives it to Lucy to play with while the others are being ground. Before she seals down the bag, she gives Lucy the opportunity to feel the soft powder and to smell its particular fragrance. Now to buy the toilet soap. There is plenty of chance to sniff and compare here, and Lucy is allowed to choose the one she likes best. Mrs B. gropes in the freezer for the fish, and then adds the bottle of lemonade to the contents of the trolley. They make for the checkout nearest the greengrocery shelves. Many of the trays for the fruit and vegetables are at the edge of the shelf, just level with Lucy's nose. Without touching them, she can feel her way along the edge of the shelf and try to identify them by smell. Here are the apples, oranges and bananas. Next come cauliflowers, onions and earthy potatoes. Each time they play this game, Lucy becomes more sure of the answers.

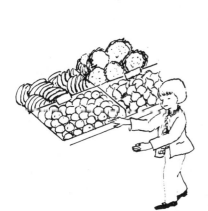

They leave the supermarket and go to the ironmongers. They find the manager arranging a new delivery of candles. He accidentally drops one. Quickly Lucy feels for it and holds it up for him. She is enjoying the sensation of wax against her hot little fingers which are rapidly exploring this fascinating object with its little tail of string. The lady who buys that candle may well wonder why it has tiny grooves all up one side!

Mrs B. buys the white spirit. The manager turns to help another customer and, while they wait to pay, Mrs B. realises she has just bought something potentially very dangerous, which is quite new to Lucy's experience. She tells her about the white spirit and that daddy will need it to clean his paint brushes. She lets her examine the bottle, then carefully removes the stopper so that she can sniff the dangerous liquid. She replaces the stopper, pays her bill and makes a great fuss of placing the bottle at the foot of the pram, well out of reach of the baby. The shopping now done, Mrs B. turns the pram towards home and a nice cup of coffee, fresh bread rolls and a refreshing drink of lemonade for Lucy.

MAKING SMELLS

Essences and perfumes can be made more manageable by sprinkling them on a small pad of cotton wool or absorbent paper. Only use a very small amount of any essence, partly to avoid waste, but mainly because strong smells — even nice ones — can sometimes give a very unpleasant sensation, for example, eucalyptus oil, if smelt too vigorously, could discourage a child from ever sniffing again! Aim at an aroma rather than a smell. An easy way of producing this is to take only one or two drops from the bottle by poking in a drinking straw just below the surface of the liquid, then hold your finger firmly over the open end. Lift the straw from the bottle, hold it over the pad you want to perfume and take your finger away. The liquid will instantly fall where you direct it. Smells can be diluted by adding them to a damp pad. To make the pad easier to handle, put it in a tin with holes in the lid or wrap it in a square of cloth and tie it in.

Smells can be sprinkled on favourite soft toys or added to fabric collage such as the Feely Trail Along the Wall (p. 150). Next time you go to a jumble or car boot sale, look out for an old-fashioned scent spray. Put in a few drops of perfume and you have a new toy! Children love to use it to squirt smelly jets of air onto their faces — good practice in squeezing too! A substitute scent spray can be made very quickly from an empty plastic detergent bottle. Take off the nozzle, wash it and thoroughly rinse out the bottle to remove all traces of the detergent smell. Cut off and throw away the stopper and the little strip of plastic that joins it to the nozzle. Put a little cotton wool or a small piece of rag impregnated with your child's favourite perfume into the bottle and replace the nozzle. The puffer makes a very satisfactory toy for most children. For the inquisitive ones, you can fix the nozzle in place with a dab of polystyrene cement — sold for making up plastic model kits. This makes the toy perfectly safe for supervised use, but will not deter a child who is really determined to remove it.

An Aromatic Herbaceous Border

Quick

Margaret Gillman
and Staff,
White Lodge Centre

In this nursery unit for children with Cerebral Palsy the staff add colour and perfume to the classroom. They make tissue paper flowers with cotton wool centres, and sprinkle them with scent. When they are not being used for decorative purposes, a child may be given one to hold, or wear as an outsized buttonhole. A child celebrating a birthday may have a garland of them draped round her wheelchair.

Each flower is made from a pipe-cleaner, a small ball of cotton wool and some tissue paper in eye-catching colours. Margaret gave me one as a sample, which I promptly vandalised to see how it was made! The dimensions given are for a flower *about* 14 cm (5½″) across. Make one to get the knack, then adjust the size as you wish.

Fold the pipe-cleaner in half. Push a cotton wool ball tightly against the bend and twist the pipe-cleaner to hold it firmly in the middle. Cut two different coloured squares of tissue paper about 14 cm square. Lay one on top of the other and pleat them together, creasing them one way and then the other, zigzag fashion, as though you were making a fan. Keeping the pleats together, fold the paper in half. With scissors, round off the corners at the open ends. Still keeping the pleats together, open out the paper and push the central crease between the ends of the pipe-cleaner and hard against the cotton wool ball. Twist up the pipe-cleaner as tightly as possible to squeeze the tissue paper and hold it in place. Tease out the pleats until each half of the flower is like a semicircular fan. Join the edges of the fans together with a dab of glue. Bend up the sharp ends of the pipe-cleaner and bind them with masking tape. Lastly, sprinkle a few drops of perfume on the cotton wool.

GAMES TO PLAY WITH SMELLY BAGS

These games are suitable for individual children or small groups.

Making Smelly Bags

Instant

Make these from squares of old material. Wrap a cotton wool ball in each square and tie it up — like a bouquet garni! Liquids can be sprinkled on the cotton wool, or powders buried inside it. If possible, involve the children in the making of the smelly bags. This way they have the opportunity of handling the substance and associating it with its smell before it disappears inside the bag.

Match the Pairs

Instant

Make up two or three pairs of bags with the same smell and invite the child to pair them off.

Spot the Stranger

Quick

Collect a few film cartons and punch holes in the lids. Make the contents of them all smell the same — except for one. You might put lavender or pot pourri in the set and a squirt of toothpaste in the 'stranger'. The possibilities are endless!

Kim's Game with Smells

Quick

Place not more than five smelly bags (with identical covers) on a tray. The child sniffs and identifies each one. He hides his eyes and one bag is removed. He must then sniff all the bags again and try to name the missing one.

Hang Out the Washing

Quick

The child pegs smelly bags at wide intervals along a low-hung washing line — the bags about level with his nose. He must then 'bring in the washing' and fetch whichever smell he is asked for.

240

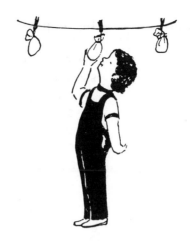

Pooh — What a Pong! Some children love to concoct *bad* smells, perhaps combining peppermint essence with vinegar! All good fun, but make sure the ingredients in the concoction are safe — albeit obnoxious! It gives children the greatest pleasure to see an adult sniff such an evil concoction and pull a face over it!

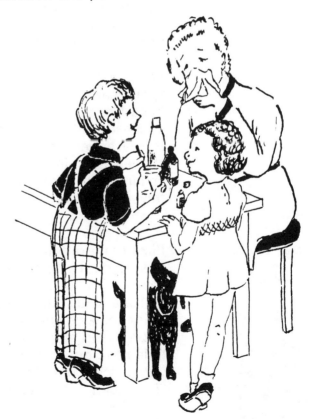

Hunt the Smell

Instant

This game is played like 'Hunt the Thimble', but a smelly bag is hidden for the child to find. (This is one occasion when you can be generous with the essence!)

All these games will only last for one session. If they are stored, all the smells will fade or combine — interesting perhaps, but useless as a scent discrimination game. One of the advantages of using film cartons is that they can be emptied and washed at the end of the session and refilled for the next time.

SMELLY GIFTS FOR CHILDREN TO MAKE

Lavender Bags

Children love making these, and they can be acceptable presents for relatives and friends. Any thin material is suitable for the bags, but one with small holes in it — like net curtaining — is nice, because the lavender can be seen inside.

The simplest lavender bag is made by putting a little pile of lavender in the centre of a square or circle of material. Gather the material round the lavender and tie up firmly with a length of ribbon. One little girl who spent many hours lying on her tummy liked to fill little bags like tiny pillow cases. She managed very well and had quite a production line going! She stripped the lavender from the stalk into a bowl. Then she shovelled it into a bag with a teaspoon, hardly spilling any. She tied up the bag with ribbon, then frayed out the top to make a decorative fringe.

Lavender Dolls

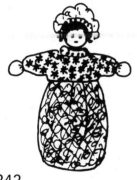

I like to make tiny brooch dolls with lavender bags as their skirts. These can be pinned to children who have severe disabilities. The child can enjoy the pleasant, delicate smell, and the brooch can serve as a talking point for any passing adult who is likely to remark upon it and stop for a chat with the child! I make a little head out of material from a pair of tights, stuffed with a scrap of polyester filling. This is inserted into a 'T'-shaped fabric torso. The skirt is made like the lavender bag above, and gathered to the torso. The features are embroidered and the head either covered with wool hair, or a little mob cap trimmed with lace. A safety pin is sewn to the back of the doll.

Pomanders

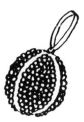

These make good Christmas presents, but need to be made in good time to allow them to dry out — so start early! Choose a well-shaped orange. Mark it vertically into four segments with narrow strips of Sellotape. This shows where the ribbon will go and defines the sections to be filled with cloves. Using a fine knitting needle, or a cocktail stick, make a hole in the orange just deep enough to take a stalk of a clove. Push in a clove, then make another hole — and so on until every section is filled. (Do not squeeze the orange or the juice may dribble out.) Roll the pomander in ground cinnamon and wrap it in foil — or waxed paper from a cereal packet. Keep it in a warm cupboard for about six weeks while it dries out and shrinks. Finally, remove the Sellotape and tie the orange up with pretty ribbon.

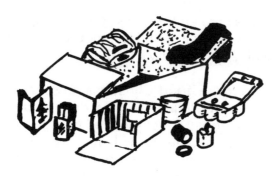

What to do with......

A CARDBOARD BOX

This is perhaps the most versatile scrap material of them all. If presented with a lovely large cardboard box, most children will instantly put their imagination to work and convert it into (in their eyes) a truly splendid toy. It can be a house, a fort, a car, boat, train, bus, or hidey hole. Turned upside down, it becomes the shell of a tortoise, the child underneath, crawling along with it on his back. With a square hole cut in one side, it is immediately transformed into a TV set ready for the child inside to present the programme. At the end of playtime, what better way of letting off steam than jumping on the box and squashing it flat!

When our children were about four and six, they saw, outside our local electrical shop, a pile of boxes put out for the dustman. A quick word with the shopkeeper, and these were soon stacked inside each other and brought home in triumph. All was ominously quiet in our son's bedroom and I went to investigate. The floor was covered with an intricate maze of cardboard boxes, their flaps raised to cover the gaps. The children were somewhere inside, happily crawling through this amazing construction!

See also
A Play Table for Bed or Floor p. 14
A Tabletop Play Corner p. 17
A Play Box, p. 17
Toss in the Bin, p. 100
Throw and Catch, p. 100
Feely Boxes — Instant and Carton p. 155
Build a Town p. 168

A SHOE BOX

- Turn it into an instant bed for a doll or teddy. A folded tea towel will do for a mattress, and a man-sized tissue for sheets. Rectangles of fabric cut with the pinking shears will pass for blankets. Collect several boxes and all the dolls and animals can go to hospital.
- Cut one or two holes in the lid, and you have a first posting box ready to receive cotton reels or square building bricks.
- Stand the box on end and cut a slot near the top of the lid to make a letter box ready to swallow a pack of playing card 'letters' — each one posted individually.
- Cut down two corners so that a long side will fold outwards and form an extension to the bottom. This can become a room for a dolls' house. Now the walls can be decorated with home-designed wall paper, the floor and its extension carpeted with fabric, windows cut out and curtains hung. Paper dolls can be cut from old magazines or dress pattern books, or more long-lasting ones concocted from pipe-cleaners and dressed in felt, or scraps of ribbon or lace.

245

Furniture can be made from matchboxes and whatever comes to hand. (When you were a child, did you ever make tiny chairs from conkers, with pins for legs, more pins for the backs and wool woven between them?) At the end of playtime, the floor extension can be folded up, the lid replaced and all the quickly made toys inside will be safely stored until next time.

See also
Smaller Feely Box p. 156
Tactile Dominoes p. 209

OTHER SMALL BOXES

- A square one makes an excellent picture cube. Stuff it with crunched-up newspaper — for extra strength — and tape it together with masking tape. Cover each face with a photograph or a picture, cut from an old Christmas card or, perhaps, a magazine. Make sure the edges of the pictures are stuck down properly or the temptation to 'pick' may be overwhelming. To make a long-lasting picture cube, cover it in clear sticky-backed plastic.
- A tea carton easily converts into a garage for a small car. Or cover it with paper and cut one long side to represent a door, add a paper fastener for a door knob, and you have a wardrobe for the shoe box dolls' house!

EGG BOXES

These have a special magic all their own. An empty box is enough to intrigue a toddler for a considerable time — just by flapping the lid, opening and closing it and feeling in all the little recesses. Later on it can be used ....

- For sorting large buttons;
- As a cash till for shop play;
- As a stacking toy. Cut out the recesses, turn them

upside down, let the children decorate them with felt pens, then pile them up one on top of the other;

● As a colour-matching game. Use two egg trays. Turn them upside down so that the recesses become mounds. Felt pens to the fore, and colour a mound on one tray and one to match it on the other. Use different colours to repeat the process (some may have to be duplicated). Cut out the mounds on one tray and, matching the colours, stack them on those of the other;

● Two mounds can be taped together with masking tape, then coloured to represent Humpty Dumpty. He can sit on the side of an egg box, ready to fall off when the punch line of the rhyme is reached.

AN ODD SOCK

● Collect a few small ones and half fill them with aquarium fish grit. Rice or dried peas are lighter, but won't wash. Sew up the top of the sock securely. Use as bean bags, or as a stacking toy — especially useful for children who find it difficult to grasp and release.

● Use longer ones as instant feely bags. Simply put a spoon or an egg cup or, perhaps, a few buttons and a marble in the toe and tie a tight knot in the leg.

● Convert one into a glove puppet (Some readers may remember Sharri Lewis and 'Lambchop'). Put the sock over your hand, and extend your fingers and thumb so that they are in opposition. Poke the tip of the toe of the sock between your fingers and thumb to make a small pocket which represents the mouth. Withdraw your hand and make a few stitches at the sides of the mouth to keep this pocket folded in. Stitch on floppy ears, eyes, nostrils, a tongue, eyebrows or whiskers .... or whatever takes your fancy.

See also
The Comet Game p. 101
Human Skittles p. 101
Sock Fights p. 101

A YOGHURT POT

- Collect several and use them as a light weight stacking and nesting toy. To make them look more elegant, the outsides can be covered with wrapping paper or scraps of Fablon.
- Use three for a 'Find It' game. Your child watches you hide a small object under one pot. He sees you change the positions of the pots, then tries to guess which one now hides the object. He lifts the pot to check if he is right. Take turns to hide the object.
- Use several pots for a target game—for children to throw or flick small objects into. The pots may need weighting for stability. A stone in each may do the trick or, for a more permanent weight, pour in a little Polyfilla and let it set.

See also
Bubble-blowing Toy p. 37
Cup and Ball Game p. 59

MATCHBOXES

- Making dolls' house furniture is an obvious way of using up a collection of matchboxes. They can rapidly be converted into beds, put together to form chunky arm chairs, dressing tables, chests of drawers, or a grandfather clock. The trays used singly can make a fireplace, or, lined with baking foil, even the kitchen sink!
- Stuff a matchbox with a tissue and cover the outside with paper or Fablon and you have a quickly-made, lightweight brick. Make lots more and a skyscraper might result.

See also
   Matchbox Pop-up p. 44
   Matchbox Puzzles p. 87

Note
Make sure the abrasive strip on the side of the box is always covered.

A PLASTIC FILM CARTON

- Put in a bell or some small buttons, glue on the lid and sew the carton into a fitting fabric bag — so that there is no possible chance the lid can be removed — and you have another noisemaker to add variety to the collection.
- Use in sand and water play. The cartons with recessed lids make excellent rollers for the sand pit and soon mark out a roadway to fit a small plastic car. Punch holes in the sides to make a mini sprinkler for water play.

See also
   A Small Pop up Dolly p. 41
   Tumbling Men p. 61
   Sound-matching Game p. 128

A STUMP OF CANDLE

- Use, as in Batik fabric printing, to make wax resistant pictures, or write secret messages. Simply use the white candle on white paper. The child then covers the paper with a wash of sloppy paint to reveal what you have drawn or written on the paper.
- Use as a washer as in the Power-driven Mobile p. 33.

A PLASTIC CARRIER BAG

- Turn one upside down, cut a head hole in the top (once the bottom) and two holes at appropriate places at the sides for arm holes and you have an instant cover-up for messy play.
- Cut round one or two in a spiral to make a *long* strip about 2 cm wide. Knit—or crochet—this (large needles or hook) to make a quick-drying and useful bag to hold the bath waterplay toys. (The printing on the bag makes a pattern as you work it in.)
- Roy's target game p. 101.

OLD CHRISTMAS CARDS

- Use them to build card towers. Choose a large and fairly stiff card for the base and stand it up as though displaying it on the mantlepiece. Lay the second card on top of it, horizontally. Stand the third card on top of that .... and so on until the skyscraper topples over.
- Use for conversation and for sorting. Together pick out all the ones with animals on, or children or snowmen ....
- Cut out the pictures carefully. Remount them to make new cards or notelets or labels for presents.

See also
Christmas Card Jigsaws p. 86
The Puzzle Game p. 97
Counting Book p. 186
Scrapbook and Tiny Scrapbook p. 186

Useful pictures
for copying

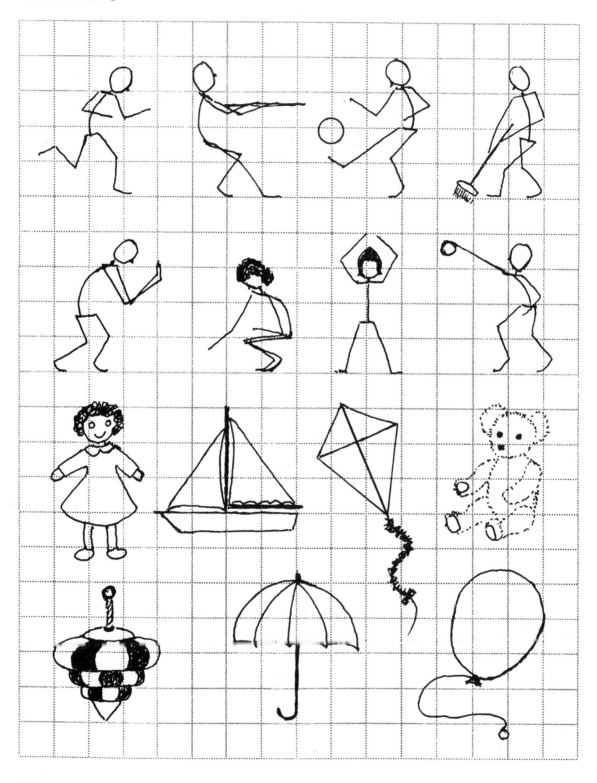

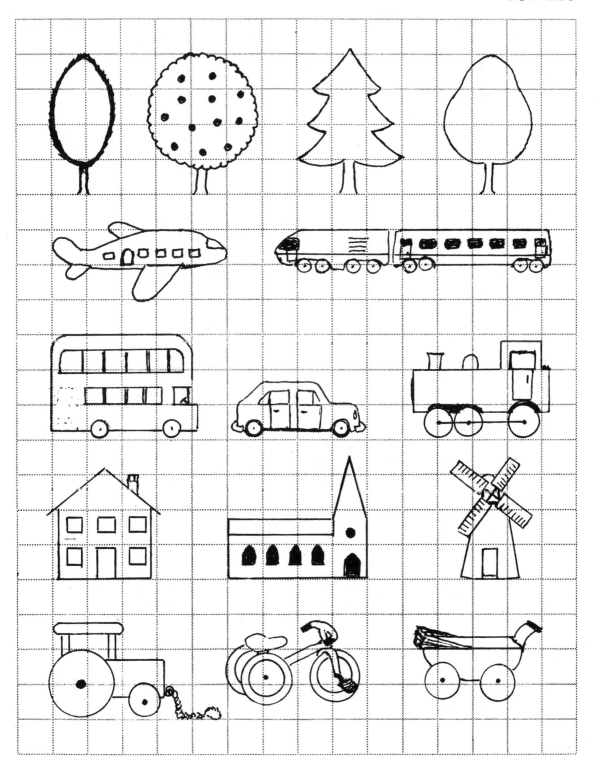

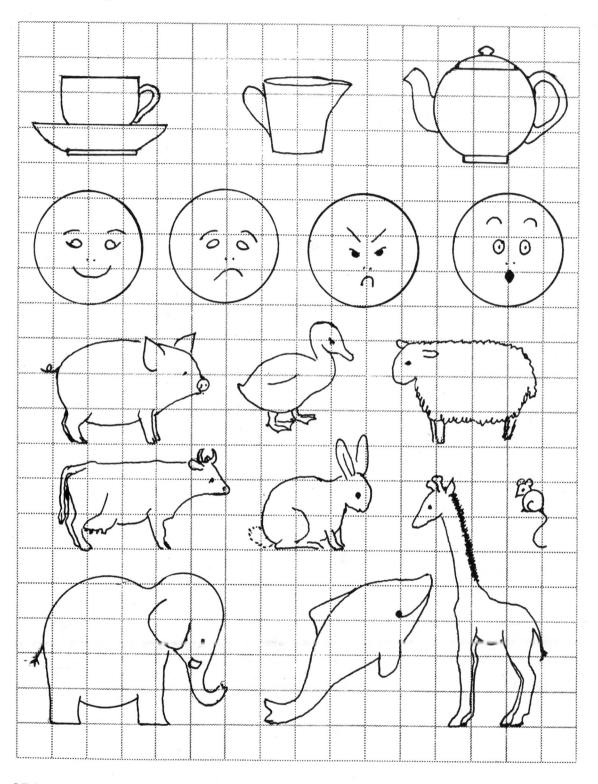

254